Common Surgical Emergencies

C. BARRIE WILLIAMS MD, FRCS
Consultant General Surgeon, City Hospital, Nottingham;
Clinical Teacher, University of Nottingham Medical School

Revised reprint

Bristol
John Wright & Sons Limited
1978

CIP Data

William, Christopher Barrie
    Common surgical emergencies/ [by] C. Barrie
    Williams. – Revised reprint.
    1. Surgery   2. Medical emergencies
    I. Title
    617'026   RD31.5

ISBN 0 7236 0501 7

Printed in Great Britain by
REDWOOD BURN LIMITED
Trowbridge & Esher

TO MY WIFE, ANN
FOR HER INFINITE PATIENCE

PREFACE

Without doubt the diagnosis of acute surgical emergencies remains a most difficult part of medicine and is, by and large, the responsibility of those in the training grades of surgery. The preliminary history taking and examination are rarely carried out under ideal conditions and yet have to be accurate so that the clinician can institute the correct treatment or start a line of investigation without delay.

I hope that this book will provide a pocket guide for students and those who have to deal with these problems; to be a reminder of important facts and instruct them in difficult basic techniques which they may have to carry out at short notice. Most of the facts are generally accepted, for if I may use a quotation of Lord Moynihan, 'I have gathered other men's posies and my contribution is the string that binds them'.

Wherever possible I have altered the text to include the helpful suggestions I received following publication of this book, and also added a section on SI units as many of the investigations required are now reported in these units. However, rare surgical emergencies such as vascular trauma have to be omitted and more specialised trauma such as fractures and head injuries deserve more space than can be accommodated here.

I am grateful to John Wright and Sons Ltd., Publishers, and particularly to Mr. A. H. B. Symons, the member of their staff who transformed my notes into proofs.

C. B. W.

Nottingham 1978

CONTENTS

Chapter 1

Patients presenting
with abdominal pain

A. PAIN DUE TO INFLAMMATION

Bacterial or chemical irritation of the abdominal cavity produces pain. The bacteria may reach the abdominal cavity from the bowel, and the chemical irritants are enzymes that have escaped from one of the digestive organs. When the inflammation is localized to the organ and its peritoneal covering a vague visceral pain is felt at the developmental site of the organ, but when the adjacent parietal peritoneum is involved pain is felt at the true anatomical position of the organ. For example, the initial visceral pain of acute appendicitis is felt in the central abdomen, but this pain later moves to the right iliac fossa as the parietal peritoneum becomes involved. In contrast, gross peritoneal contamination following a perforated peptic ulcer or acute pancreatitis produces a sudden pain affecting most, if not all, of the abdomen.

As well as local symptoms and signs more general effects such as sweating, nausea, vomiting, tachycardia, and pyrexia accompany intra-abdominal inflammations.

ACUTE APPENDICITIS

Acute appendicitis is the commonest condition encountered in general surgery and during the past 30 years there has been a real improvement in its diagnosis and treatment. This is evident from the *Registrar-General's*

Statistical Review of England and Wales which revealed for the years 1940, 1950, 1960 and 1970 a progressive fall in the mortality of acute appendicitis of 2378, 1299, 638 and 327 respectively.

SYMPTOMS

i. *Anorexia.*

ii. *Pain.* Umbilical, later moving to the right iliac fossa.

iii. *Nausea.* May vomit once or occasionally twice during the early stages.

iv. Diarrhoea (retro-ileal appendix).

v. Frequency of micturition (pelvic appendix).

vi. Flexion of the right thigh (retrocaecal appendix).

SIGNS

i. *Furred tongue and foetor oris.*

ii. *Pain* in the right iliac fossa when coughing.

iii. *Tenderness and guarding* in the right iliac fossa with rebound tenderness later.

iv. Steadily increasing pulse-rate.

v. Hyperaesthesia over the right iliac fossa.

vi. Tenderness on rectal examination.

INVESTIGATIONS

Specific tests for any differential diagnosis that may be considered.

DIFFERENTIAL DIAGNOSIS

Almost all acute abdominal conditions and some thoracic conditions may be considered in the differential diagnosis of acute appendicitis as occasionally the diagnosis can be extremely difficult. However, it must be remembered that acute appendicitis is so common that it may occur with any other surgical condition.

Acute appendicitis during pregnancy is often atypical as the appendix is displaced upwards by the uterus. This can lead to delay in diagnosis particularly if, as is often the case, the symptoms are considered to be due to pyelitis. If acute appendicitis is even suspected during pregnancy an appendicectomy should be carried out.

TREATMENT

   i. Appendicectomy.

   ii. Antibiotics when peritonitis is present.

APPENDIX MASS

When acute appendicitis progresses untreated the adjacent structures and omentum surround the appendix and wall it off from the general peritoneal cavity by forming fibrous adhesions. This localization of the infection usually leads to resolution of the inflammation but may produce an abscess containing pus and a necrotic appendix.

SYMPTOMS

   i. History of acute appendicitis 3–7 days previously.

   ii. Anorexia.

SIGNS

   i. *Tender mass*, usually in the right iliac fossa, but its site varies with the position of the appendix. A pelvic appendix mass may be felt rectally.

INVESTIGATIONS

   i. White blood-count elevated.

   ii. Haemoglobin level may be reduced.

DIFFERENTIAL DIAGNOSIS

There is usually no difficulty in making the diagnosis but carcinoma of the caecum, regional ileitis, actinomycosis, and a twisted ovarian cyst may have to be excluded.

TREATMENT

a. Conservative Treatment (Ochsner–Sherren Régime)
This is only carried out when no doubt exists about the diagnosis and the patients are aged between 10 and 65 years when the normal body defences can be depended upon.

i. Nasogastric aspiration.

ii. Intravenous fluids.

iii. Hourly measurement of the pulse-rate and 4-hourly measurement of the temperature.

iv. The size of the mass is measured and its outline drawn on the patient's abdomen. The abdomen is checked regularly for changes in size of the mass.

v. Analgesics. These are not usually required, particularly after the first 6–12 hours.

vi. No antibiotics are given as they mask the signs used to gauge the success of conservative treatment.

b. Surgical Treatment
Conservative treatment must be stopped and surgery carried out when there is:

i. Persistent pain.

ii. Rising pulse-rate. Compared with this, changes in the temperature are relatively unimportant although a swinging temperature is a late sign of abscess formation requiring surgery.

iii. Increase in size of the mass.

iv. Abscess formation.

v. Peritonitis.

vi. Intestinal obstruction.

The majority of patients with an appendix mass settle with conservative treatment and appendicectomy is carried out some 6–12 weeks later. If the régime is abandoned for any of the above reasons then antibiotics are given and drainage of the abscess, with or without appendicectomy, is carried out.

ACUTE CHOLECYSTITIS

Acute cholecystitis invariably occurs in the presence of gall-stones, and when the cystic duct becomes blocked by a stone or oedema the inflammatory products are unable to escape from the gall-bladder and remain to form an empyema. Rare complications of acute cholecystitis are gangrene of the gall-bladder and perforation of its wall to produce a biliary peritonitis.

SYMPTOMS

i. *Pain* in the right hypochondrium and back. It is either constant or of increasing severity.

ii. *Nausea and vomiting*.

iii. Past history of flatulent dyspepsia and fatty intolerance.

iv. Rigors.

SIGNS

i. *Pyrexia*.

ii. *Tenderness and guarding* over the gall-bladder area.

iii. An oedematous gall-bladder may be felt but this is usually obscured by rigidity of the abdominal wall.

iv. Hyperaesthesia over the angles of the ninth to eleventh ribs on the right.

v. Slight jaundice.

INVESTIGATIONS

i. White blood-count significantly raised.

ii. Urea and serum electrolytes if vomiting is persistent.

iii. Liver-function tests on serum.

iv. X-rays. (*a*) Straight X-ray of abdomen will show gall-stones in 10 per cent of cases. (*b*) Oral cholecystography either on admission or when the inflammatory episode has settled. In the former case non-visualization of the gall-bladder is open to so many interpretations that it is valueless, but a functioning gall-bladder means that an incorrect diagnosis has been made.

v. Haemoglobin and cross-match 2 units of blood if surgery is considered during the acute phase.

TREATMENT

a. *Conservative Treatment*

This method of treatment is used by the majority of clinicians and aims at allowing the inflammation to settle completely so that a cholecystectomy can be carried out under optimum conditions at a later date.

i. Nasogastric aspiration.

ii. Intravenous fluids.

iii. Analgesics, e.g., pethidine.

iv. Antibiotics. Tetracycline is the antibiotic of choice as not only does it reach the wall of the gall-bladder via the blood-stream but it is also excreted in the bile. It is given intramuscularly during the acute phase and as tablets once the patient can tolerate oral medication.

In the majority of cases conservative management is successful but it must be abandoned in favour of surgery if:

i. The diagnosis is in doubt.

ii. The pulse-rate is rising after 24 hours of treatment.

iii. The pain is spreading.

iv. An empyema of the gall-bladder forms. This is diagnosed by the presence of a painful tender mass in the right hypochondrium with an increasing pulse-rate and swinging temperature.

v. The gall-bladder perforates. This causes a rapid and profound toxaemia with a rising pulse-rate and temperature. There is generalized tenderness with guarding and rebound tenderness.

vi. Diabetic patient out of control.

vii. The patient is pregnant.

b. Surgical Treatment

Surgery as the primary treatment of choice is advised by a minority of surgeons as several large series have shown no difference in morbidity and mortality when conservative treatment with delayed cholecystectomy is compared with immediate surgery. However, they stress that an immediate operation must be performed by an experienced surgeon. Either a cholecystectomy with an operative cholangiogram or a cholecystostomy removing all the stones and draining the gall-bladder is carried out. The choice of procedure depends upon the condition of the patient and inclination of the surgeon.

ACUTE PANCREATITIS

This is an autodigestion of the pancreas which produces oedema and haemorrhage in the organ and allows pancreatic enzymes to escape into the retroperitoneal tissues, peritoneal cavity and blood-stream. Here they produce both local and generalized effects. The aetiology is obscure. Approximately one-half of the cases are associated with gall-stones but others occur with alcoholic cirrhosis or following abdominal operations. In about one-third of cases no aetiological factor is found. The condition is relatively benign in patients less than 50 years old, but carries a high mortality in the elderly and when trauma or steroids play a part in the aetiology. Apart from the initial shock the factors which contribute to the mortality rate are progressive respiratory or renal failure. As the condition settles necrosis of the pancreas may occur with the formation of abscesses and pseudocysts.

SYMPTOMS

   i. *Pain*, of sudden onset in the upper abdomen and radiating to the back. Later the pain may become generalized.

   ii. *Persistent vomiting and retching*, either the result of obstruction of the duodenum by oedema of the head of the pancreas or of irritation of the coeliac ganglion by the escaping enzymes.

SIGNS

i. *Shock*. Shock which is often profound is produced by exudation of large amounts of plasma, red blood cell destruction and the release into the blood-stream of vasoactive substances such as kallikrein and bradykinin. The patient is pale or even cyanotic, cold, and sweating with hypotension and a weak pulse. The temperature is initially subnormal but rises later.

ii. *Epigastric tenderness* and in the majority of patients tenderness is also found over the tail of the pancreas at the left costovertebral angle.

iii. Muscle rigidity over the abdomen (less than 50 per cent of patients).

iv. Jaundice (less than 20 per cent of patients). This is usually a late sign caused by cholangitis, obstruction of the common bile-duct by a stone, or the oedematous head of the pancreas.

INVESTIGATIONS

i. *Serum amylase*. This quickly rises to reach the highest levels 5–12 hours after the onset of the attack and then falls rapidly to reach a normal level within 48 hours. The normal range is 80–180 Somogyi units per 100 ml. or 3–10 Wohlgemuth units per 1 ml. Serum levels in excess of 1000 Somogyi units per 100 ml. are very strongly suggestive of acute pancreatitis and only blood levels of at least 500 Somogyi units per 100 ml. or 100 Wohlgemuth units per 1 ml. are considered significant. Thirty per cent of patients with acute pancreatitis have normal serum amylase levels.

ii. Urine amylase. During the first 24 hours of an

attack of acute pancreatitis very high values are reached and then the level slowly falls to normal over a period of 7–10 days. The normal excretion rate is 8000–30,000 Wohlgemuth units per 24 hours (average 2–50 Wohlgemuth units per ml.).

iii. White blood-count elevated to 10,000–30,000 per c.mm.

iv. Serum calcium. The serum calcium level tends to fall during the course of the illness but in the majority of cases it remains above the lower limit of the normal range. It can be a guide to the severity of the condition as the lower the result the more severe tends to be the illness. The fall may be partly due to calcium combining with the free fatty acids released by digestion, but other factors such as the effects of glucagon or a low serum albumin may play an important role.

v. Abdominal X-ray. This may show gall-stones or a 'sentinel loop' due to gaseous distension of the duodenum, transverse colon, or small bowel.

DIFFERENTIAL DIAGNOSIS

This may be difficult and the following must be considered: cholecystitis and biliary colic, perforated peptic ulcer, appendicitis in a high position, mesenteric infarction, and coronary thrombosis. Great reliance is placed on the measurement of serum amylase but this may be elevated, although not to such a high level, in biliary disease, perforated peptic ulceration, strangulation of intestine, renal failure, and after opiates have been given. When the diagnosis is difficult an early laparotomy has been advocated as the operation does not seem to increase the mortality of acute pancreatitis now that the nature of the associated shock is understood. A laparotomy will prevent the clinician from missing diagnoses such as strangulation obstruction of the intestine where incorrect treatment can be fatal.

TREATMENT

The initial treatment of acute pancreatitis is conservative but surgery may be required later to treat the various complications.

i. *Nasogastric aspiration.* This relieves the retching and prevents gastric content from entering the duodenum and releasing the hormones that stimulate the pancreas.

ii. *Intravenous fluids.* Large quantities of fluid which are lost into the retroperitoneal space and peritoneal cavity must be replaced. Plasma or whole blood may be required to correct blood-loss if hypotension persists in spite of giving clear intravenous fluids. Measurement of the central venous pressure (C.V.P.) is invaluable for controlling the amount of fluid required.

iii. *Analgesics.* Regular doses of pethidine are given intravenously, or intramuscularly when the peripheral circulation is adequate for absorption. Morphine and opiates must not be used as they produce spasm of the sphincter of Oddi, thereby worsening the condition.

iv. *Antispasmodics.* Propantheline bromide (Pro-Banthine) intravenously every 6 hours reduces pancreatic secretion and relaxes the sphincter of Oddi.

v. Calcium gluconate: 10 mg. in a 10 per cent solution either intravenously or intramuscularly every 24–48 hours if the serum calcium remains low.

vi. Isoprenaline (monitored by continuous E.C.G. tracing) when hypotension persists in spite of fluid replacement.

vii. Trasylol (FBA Pharmaceuticals Ltd.), a proteolytic enzyme inhibitor active against trypsin and kallikrein, has had variable clinical results but does appear to reduce the high mortality rate for patients over 50 years of age.

viii. Glucagon, which is isolated from crude preparations of insulin, has an unclear place in the treatment of acute pancreatitis but does produce a dramatic relief of pain in a number of patients.

ix. Steroids. The use of corticosteroids is also controversial but in severe cases they may be used to reduce the inflammatory response.

x. Antibiotics may be used when secondary infection is suspected.

A poor prognosis is associated with persistently raised white blood-counts and serum fibrinogen levels or a persistently low serum calcium (less than 7 mg. per 100 ml.).

SIGMOID DIVERTICULITIS

In sigmoid diverticulosis the mucosa of the sigmoid colon protrudes between its taeniae coli to form sacs where stasis and infection can occur. When infection occurs the bowel wall becomes thickened and tender. Adjacent loops of small intestine may become involved in the inflammatory mass to produce a picture of intestinal obstruction. Perforation of a diverticulum into the peritoneal cavity or haemorrhage into the lumen of the bowel can also occur.

SYMPTOMS

i. *Pain.* This is a constant pain in the left iliac fossa and hypogastric region.

ii. *Change in bowel habit.* Although it may be either constipation or diarrhoea there is usually a more recent history of constipation.

iii. Nausea and vomiting.

iv. A single profuse haemorrhage per rectum.

SIGNS

i. *Pyrexia.*

ii. *Tenderness in the left iliac fossa.*

iii. Tenderness and warmth to the left on rectal examination.

iv. Palpable mass in the left iliac fossa (30 per cent of patients).

INVESTIGATIONS
i. White blood-count elevated.
ii. Barium-enema examination must be deferred until the inflammation has settled.

DIFFERENTIAL DIAGNOSIS
There is usually no difficulty in diagnosis.

TREATMENT
The initial treatment is conservative but immediate surgery is required for complications such as perforation, intestinal obstruction, abscess formation, and persistent severe haemorrhage. Fistulae into the small intestine and bladder or stenosis of the colon may require surgery when the active phase has settled.
i. *Bed-rest.*
ii. *Analgesics.* Both pethidine and pentazocine hydrochloride (Fortral) are useful in this condition.
iii. *Broad-spectrum antibiotics.*
iv. Low-roughage diet. This is given until the inflammation has settled and then a high-roughage diet is recommended.
v. Antispasmodics. Propantheline bromide may be given but it can precipitate urinary retention in the elderly.

PERFORATED PEPTIC ULCER
Eighty per cent of perforations occur in chronic peptic ulcers and 20 per cent in acute peptic ulcers or gastric neoplasms. Patients with acute ulcers often give a history of recent stress or the ingestion of substances known to irritate the stomach wall, e.g., aspirin and phenylbutazone. In the vast majority of cases the ulcer perforates into either the greater or lesser sacs of the peritoneal cavity and the subsequent course of events can be roughly divided into three stages. However, difficulty in diagnosis may occur when a small perforation is quickly sealed off.

The first stage of *peritonism* begins with a sudden onset of pain and is the result of peritoneal irritation by acid from the stomach. It lasts for 3–6 hours. During the second stage of *reaction* the acid is neutralized by a copious outpouring of peritoneal fluid and the patient feels better. This stage lasts 3–6 hours and is followed by the third stage of *peritonitis* when bacterial invasion of the peritoneal cavity occurs. At this point the patient's condition begins to deteriorate rapidly if he has not been treated. The mortality of this condition increases with the age of the patient and the length of time between the perforation and treatment.

SYMPTOMS AND SIGNS (*Table* 1)

Table 1. SYMPTOMS AND SIGNS OF PERFORATED PEPTIC ULCERATION

	STAGE		
	I	II	III
Symptoms			
Abdominal pain	Severe; sudden onset	Eases	Increases
Shoulder-tip pain	±	+	+
Vomiting	±	+	+ + +
Shock	+ +	+	+ +
Signs			
Temperature	Subnormal	Normal	Variable
Pulse	Normal	Normal or rising	Rapid and small volume
Abdominal rigidity	+ + +	+ +	+
Abdominal distension	−	−	+ +
Bowel-sounds	±	−	−
Respirations	Shallow	Shallow and thoracic; ala nasi working	Laboured and rapid
Liver dullness	Present	Diminished	Absent
Tenderness p.r.	−	+	+

INVESTIGATIONS

i. Haemoglobin and packed-cell volume ⎱
ii. Serum electrolytes and urea ⎰ These results give an idea as to the degree of dehydration.

iii. White blood-count, rises in the third stage.

iv. Cross-match 4 units of blood if major gastric surgery is anticipated.

v. *X-ray abdomen.* Gas under the diaphragm is seen on the erect film in 70 per cent of cases.

DIFFERENTIAL DIAGNOSIS

This includes coronary thrombosis, acute pancreatitis, acute cholecystitis, biliary colic, basal pneumonia, and acute appendicitis which is often simulated by a perforated duodenal ulcer that has leaked along the right paracolic gutter.

TREATMENT

This is usually surgical although a conservative régime may be the choice in certain circumstances, e.g., absence of operating facilities and medical contra-indications to surgery. For both forms of treatment the initial management is the same:

i. Analgesics, e.g., morphine.
ii. Broad-spectrum antibiotics.
iii. Nasogastric aspiration.
iv. Intravenous fluids.

a. Surgical Treatment

This includes peritoneal lavage with warm saline and either simple suturing of the perforation or a definitive procedure. The type of operation carried out will depend upon the experience of the surgeon, age and condition of the patient, and the length of time since perforation.

b. Conservative Treatment

Patients with acute ulceration or patients who because of

associated disease are considered unfit for operation may be treated with a conservative régime.

i. Analgesics. Morphine 15 mg. subcutaneously—only one dose may be given.

ii. Continuous nasogastric aspiration. This must be regularly checked at least every 30 minutes.

iii. Intravenous fluids.

iv. Antibiotics.

v. Regular monitoring of the pulse (every half-hour), blood-pressure (every hour), temperature (every 4 hours), and an accurate fluid balance chart must be kept.

Conservative management is abandoned in favour of surgery when:

i. Doubt exists about the diagnosis.

ii. More than one dose of morphine is required to alleviate the pain which should be very much improved within 6 hours of starting treatment.

iii. The patient has recently ingested a heavy meal.

iv. Bleeding as well as perforation is present.

v. Pyloric stenosis is present.

vi. The pulse-rate is steadily rising.

ACUTE SALPINGITIS

The causative organisms of acute salpingitis include gono-coccus, streptococcus, *Escherichia coli*, and pneumococcus. Material formed in the infected Fallopian tubes may either escape into the peritoneal cavity and vagina or remain in the tube to form an abscess (pyosalpinx). The abscess may later rupture into the peritoneal cavity. Acute salpingitis may also arise soon after an abortion or normal delivery.

SYMPTOMS

i. *Pain*, which is constant and low in the iliac fossae.

ii. *Purulent vaginal discharge*.

iii. Nausea or vomiting.

iv. Recent menstrual irregularities.

v. Frequency of micturition (common).

vi. Dysuria (rare).

SIGNS

i. *Pyrexia.*

ii. *Bilateral low tenderness* over the iliac fossae with or without guarding.

iii. *Pelvic tenderness and warmth* on rectal or vaginal examination.

INVESTIGATIONS

i. White blood-count, in excess of 12,000 per c.mm.

ii. E.S.R., elevated.

iii. Haemoglobin, sometimes reduced.

iv. Microscopy and culture of a fresh specimen of the vaginal discharge.

v. Serology for gonococcus and syphilis.

TREATMENT

i. *Antibiotics.* Tetracycline is the antibiotic of choice either intramuscularly or orally if the patient is not vomiting. The antibiotic is changed if the sensitivities show that the organism is resistant to tetracycline. Streptomycin must not be given until tuberculosis has been excluded.

ii. Correction of anaemia with either iron or blood.

iii. Surgery when a pyosalpinx or generalized peritonitis is present.

SMALL INTESTINAL DIVERTICULITIS

When present, diverticula of the jejunum are found on the mesenteric border of the bowel and vary in both number and size. They have been associated with flatulence and malabsorption syndromes such as anaemia, steatorrhoea, hypoproteinaemia, and avitaminosis. They may also produce vague epigastric pains that radiate down the left side of the abdomen.

Meckel's diverticula are reputed to be present in 2 per cent of the population, situated 60 cm. (2 ft.) from the ileocaecal junction and are approximately 5 cm. (2 in.) long. Symptoms may result from: (*a*) inflammation of its wall, (*b*) peptic ulceration or haemorrhage as it may contain gastric mucosa, (*c*) intestinal obstruction by a fibrous band that sometimes runs from its tip to the umbilicus or when it forms the apex of an intussusception.

The diverticula may produce symptoms and signs similar to acute appendicitis and are usually diagnosed at laparotomy. The treatment is surgical, removing the inflamed diverticulum.

B. PAIN DUE TO OBSTRUCTION

When a hollow organ attempts to deal with a partial or complete obstruction of its lumen it produces vigorous peristaltic contractions which give rise to colicky pains. The pain is felt either as visceral pain at the site of embryological origin of the organ, or as referred pain at a part of the body sharing the same nerve-supply. For example, pain produced by a stone in the ureter may be referred to the penis, scrotum, and top of the thigh, all of which are supplied by the nerves T.10 to L.1.

During each spasm of pain the patient rolls about trying to find a position that will give some relief, and between pains the patient relaxes waiting for the next one.

The pain may be accompanied by vomiting which varies in volume and frequency according to its cause. In intestinal obstruction the volume of vomit may be great and its appearance depends upon the level of the obstruction. The initial acid stomach content will be followed by bile or bile-stained small intestinal matter and later, though very rarely, by faeculent material originating in the large intestine.

In other forms of colic where vomiting is not the result of attempts to overcome intestinal obstruction the vomiting is a reflex action. The vomit then consists of small amounts of material which, once the stomach is empty, become infrequent and only consist of saliva or gastric juice.

BILIARY COLIC

Biliary colic occurs when stones formed in the gall-bladder obstruct the cystic duct. If the stone causes a complete obstruction a mucocele results as mucus produced by the gall-bladder is unable to escape. The stone may pass through the duct and obstruct the common bile-duct, producing jaundice.

SYMPTOMS

i. *Colic* in the right hypochondrium, epigastrium, and referred pain in an area just below the angle of the right scapula.

ii. *Retching* and vomiting of small amounts.

iii. May give a history of flatulent dyspepsia and fat intolerance.

SIGNS

None of note.

INVESTIGATIONS

At a convenient time the white blood-count and liver-function tests on the serum should be measured to act as base lines during future management.

X-rays

i. Straight abdomen. Only 10 per cent of gall-stones are radio-opaque, but the X-ray can be used to exclude a perforated peptic ulcer if it is considered in the differential diagnosis.

ii. Cholecystogram. This should be left for 3 or 4 days as liver function is depressed during the acute episode.

DIFFERENTIAL DIAGNOSIS

The diagnosis is not usually difficult, but acute cholecystitis, acute pancreatitis, and a leaking peptic ulcer must be excluded.

TREATMENT

a. Conservative Treatment

i. Analgesics, e.g., pethidine. Morphine and opiates must be avoided.

ii. Antispasmodics, e.g., propantheline bromide orally, or subcutaneously if vomiting is present.

iii. Fat-free diet.

b. Surgical Treatment

A cholecystectomy is carried out at any time after admission depending upon the policy of the surgeon in charge. It is worth while checking that facilities for operative cholangiography are available.

MECHANICAL INTESTINAL OBSTRUCTION

Obstruction can occur at any point along the alimentary tract and the causative pathology tends to vary with the site. For example, while adhesions, bands, and external herniae are by far the commonest obstructing factors in the small intestine, the majority of large-bowel obstructions are the result of cancer. The symptoms and signs produced depend on the level and completeness of the obstruction and whether or not strangulation of the bowel is present.

SYMPTOMS AND SIGNS

Because the rate of onset of symptoms in small-bowel obstructions is more rapid than large-bowel lesions they are often referred to as acute and chronic obstructions respectively (*Table* 2).

It is important to decide early whether or not strangulation of the bowel has occurred as this determines the type of treatment required. Fortunately most patients with strangulation present dramatically and although the signs are often indefinite the following can help:

   i. Continuous pain rather than colic.
   ii. Localized guarding and tenderness with rebound.
   iii. Rising pulse-rate and temperature.
   iv. Early shock.
   v. Leucocytosis.

Table 2. SYMPTOMS AND SIGNS IN NON-STRANGULATED INTESTINAL OBSTRUCTION

	SMALL INTESTINE	LARGE INTESTINE
Colic	Epigastric or umbilical; the higher the obstruction the more frequent the pains	Hypogastric The pain may be delayed in onset or even absent
Vomiting	Early	Infrequent and late
Constipation	Late	Early
Abdominal distension	Late, slight or absent	Early
Shock and dehydration	Early	Insignificant
Scars on the abdomen or hernia present	Significant	Not usually significant
Visible loops of bowel with peristalsis	Significant	Significant
Increased bowel-sounds	Present	Present

INVESTIGATIONS

   i. Haemoglobin and packed-cell volume.
   ii. Serum electrolytes and urea.
   iii. Urine output, specific gravity, and electrolytes.
   iv. Central venous pressure measurement. This helps

in the assessment of dehydration and is useful when replacing fluid loss, particularly in the elderly and patients where the cardiac state is doubtful.

v. X-rays. Erect and supine of the abdomen. The erect or decubitus (when the patient is unable to sit up) films will show fluid levels in the bowel proximal to the obstruction. The pattern of the distended bowel may also give a rough idea as to the level of the obstruction. Valvulae conniventes can be seen as parallel lines crossing the full width of the jejunum and proximal ileum whereas the terminal ileum appears characterless. The large-bowel haustrations are more widely spaced and do not pass across the complete width of the lumen.

Less commonly impacted faecal masses can be seen, a gall-stone is identified outside the area of the gall-bladder, or the typical large dilated sigmoid loop of a volvulus is apparent.

vi. Two-enema test. In doubtful cases this test helps to confirm a complete colonic obstruction. The first enema often produces a faecal result but a second enema performed a couple of hours later produces neither faeces nor flatus.

DIFFERENTIAL DIAGNOSIS

When distension is absent one must consider acute inflammatory conditions, perforations, and acute pancreatitis, and when distension is present uraemia, mesenteric thrombosis, and peritonitis must be excluded.

TREATMENT

In the majority of cases it is worth while spending a couple of hours preparing the patient for operation. But the timing of any surgery will depend upon the cause of the obstruction, the state of the patient, and whether or not further improvement in the state of the patient can be anticipated.

i. *Intravenous fluids.* The amount of fluid and electrolytes required to correct the dehydration must be estimated and progress during replacement checked with C.V.P. measurements and repeated packed-cell volume and electrolyte estimations. An accurate chart of fluid input and urinary output is essential. Blood or plasma is required when strangulation or peritonitis is present.

ii. *Nasogastric aspiration.*

iii. Antibiotics. These are required either when peritonitis is present, e.g., tetracycline, or if resection of the large bowel is planned at a later date, e.g., neomycin or phthalylsulphathiazole.

iv. Analgesics.

v. When a sigmoid volvulus is present an attempt can be made to decompress the sigmoid colon by passing a well-lubricated, wide, plastic oesophageal tube into the sigmoid colon through a sigmoidoscope that has been introduced to the rectosigmoid junction.

vi. *Surgery.* An immediate operation is required with the least preparation of the patient when:

a. Strangulation of the bowel is present.

b. Mesenteric vascular occlusion is present.

c. When there is deterioration in the patient's condition or failure to improve in spite of resuscitative measures.

d. When the pulse-rate rises or fails to settle.

RENAL PAIN AND URETERIC COLIC

Renal pain is the constant pain felt in the loin when there is distension or irritation of the kidney and renal pelvis. Ureteric pain is a colic produced by peristalsis of the ureter attempting to overcome an obstruction of its lumen. The commonest cause of ureteric obstruction is a urinary calculus, but other conditions producing colic include the passage of blood, debris, or pus and the kinking of the ureter of a mobile kidney.

SYMPTOMS

   i. *Colic* at any position in a line from the loin to the penis, testicle, or thigh.

   ii. *Retching* or vomiting small amounts.

   iii. Haematuria, although this is usually microscopic.

SIGNS

Usually there are none but occasionally a tender or enlarged kidney can be felt.

INVESTIGATIONS

   i. *Microscopy of the urine.* Immediate examination of the deposit of a centrifuged specimen of urine reveals red blood-cells. The deposit should be cultured for bacterial growth.

   ii. *X-rays.*

   a. A straight X-ray demonstrates the stone in 80–90 per cent of patients. The stone is seen along the line of the ureter which runs along the tips of the transverse processes from L.1 to L.5 and then passes across the sacro-iliac joint towards the ischial spine before turning medially towards the pubic tubercle.

   b. Excretion urography (I.V.P.) is invaluable and should be carried out on admission whenever possible. It may show delayed function, a swollen nephrogram, and the site and size of the stone. It also confirms the state and function of the other kidney.

   iii. Serum calcium, phosphate, and uric acid estimations.

   iv. Analysis of the stone when it is available.

DIFFERENTIAL DIAGNOSIS

This can be difficult but when an excretory urogram is carried out the diagnosis is quickly confirmed.

TREATMENT

The majority of cases of ureteric calculus respond to

conservative management which includes:

    i. *High fluid intake.* At least 3 litres a day.

    ii. *Analgesics.* Although not as potent as the opiates, pethidine is preferred as it produces much less muscular spasm.

    iii. Antispasmodics. Their usefulness is questionable as they may interfere with the peristalsis required for the patient to pass the stone spontaneously.

    Surgery is only indicated when:

    i. The urine is infected.

    ii. The stone is obviously too large to pass.

    iii. Repeated attacks of colic occur with no advancement of the stone.

    iv. There is complete obstruction of the ureter with back pressure on the kidney.

    When surgery is required the stone is usually removed by ureterotomy, but if the stone is in the lowest inch of the ureter extraction with a Dormia basket can be attempted by a surgeon skilled in its use.

C. PAIN DUE TO ISCHAEMIA

MESENTERIC INFARCTION

This uncommon cause of intestinal obstruction results from an acute blockage of the mesenteric blood-vessels by thrombosis or embolus. It is associated with a very high mortality and the single most important factor in the survival of these patients is early diagnosis. Unfortunately, the condition has few signs during the early stages and once gangrene with peritonitis has occurred the diagnosis is relatively simple but the prognosis is very poor.

    The area of infarction and hence the seriousness of the condition varies with the size and position of the occluded vessel. The superior mesenteric vessels are involved more often than the inferior ones which also have a better collateral circulation. The bowel soon becomes paralysed and haemorrhagic. At the same time blood is poured into the lumen of the bowel and a blood-stained peritoneal exudate is produced. This results in a considerable loss of blood-volume with a fall in systolic blood-pressure and a state of collapse closely resembling an internal haemorrhage. The bowel distends, develops an ileus, and peritonitis soon follows.

The origin of the embolus may be the mitral valve, left auricular appendage (both usually in patients with chronic rheumatic heart disease), or an atheromatous plaque on the aorta. Thrombosis in the mesenteric vessels may be the result of atherosclerosis, poor cardiac output, hypotensive disorders, thrombo-angiitis obliterans, portal hypertension, and pyelophlebitis. Patients with a mesenteric infarction therefore often have a serious underlying disease which will adversely affect the prognosis.

SYMPTOMS

i. *Severe abdominal pain.* Usually of sudden onset, poorly localized and unresponsive to narcotics.

ii. Repeated vomiting.

iii. Diarrhoea.

iv. Tenesmus.

v. Past history of rheumatic heart disease, atherosclerosis, etc.

SIGNS

i. Pallor.

ii. Hypotension.

iii. Auricular fibrillation.

iv. Atherosclerosis.

v. Ill-defined mass, palpable in the abdomen.

vi. Blood or blood-stained stool in the rectum.

vii. Abdominal rigidity. This occurs late and first develops over the affected bowel. It becomes generalized as peritonitis progresses.

viii. Abdominal distension is also a late sign.

INVESTIGATIONS

i. Haemoglobin and packed-cell volume.

ii. Serum electrolytes and urea.

iii. White blood-count is elevated.

iv. Group and cross-match 2–4 units of blood.

v. Serum amylase is elevated, but not to the levels found in acute pancreatitis.

vi. X-ray abdomen. Multiple small-bowel loops with fluid levels soon develop with the translucent areas separated by thickened oedematous bowel wall.

vii. Diagnostic abdominal paracentesis reveals blood-stained peritoneal fluid.

DIFFERENTIAL DIAGNOSIS

Among the many diagnoses to be considered are acute pancreatitis, internal haemorrhage, dissecting aneurysm, perforations, and coronary thrombosis.

TREATMENT

i. Intravenous fluids. Plasma or dextran are used to replace the fluid lost and blood is needed to replace the blood-loss.

ii. Nasogastric aspiration.

iii. Antibiotics, e.g., kanamycin or cephaloridine.

iv. Treatment of any cardiac failure or arrhythmia.

v. Oxygen.

vi. Anticoagulants, e.g., heparin to prevent the further spread of thrombosis.

vii. Immediate surgery either resecting the involved bowel or by embolectomy if a long length of intestine is involved.

Chapter 2

Patients presenting with acute blood-loss

Table 3 provides a rough guide when estimating blood-loss but each individual sign must be considered with any other signs that may be present. For example, the blood-pressure can be maintained at a normal level in an otherwise fit patient even when quite severe blood-loss

Table 3. PATIENTS PRESENTING WITH ACUTE BLOOD-LOSS

DEGREE OF BLOOD-LOSS	BODY RESPONSE AND EFFECTS	SYMPTOMS AND SIGNS
Mild <25% of blood-volume	Generalized peripheral vasoconstriction in the kidney, skin, and mesentery; this directs the available blood to important sites	May be heralded by faintness; pallor
Moderate 25–50% of blood-volume	The cardiac output is increased to maintain the blood-pressure	Pulse-rate increased; pulse volume low (thready); hypotension; cold clammy skin; empty veins; anxiety and restlessness
Severe 50%+ of blood-volume	Anoxia of the C.N.S.	Thirst; deep sighing respirations (air hunger); tinnitus; blindness

has occurred, but other signs will be present to warn the clinician. Acute blood-loss in children and elderly patients presents particular problems. In children the loss of a small amount of blood may represent a large proportion of the total blood-volume and, because the peripheral resistance is normally high in children, compensation by vasoconstriction is greatly limited. The atherosclerotic arteries of elderly patients hinder responses to any blood-loss and jeopardizes an already impaired circulation to the brain and heart.

INVESTIGATIONS

i. Haemoglobin. When no treatment is forthcoming an acute blood-loss is followed within a few hours by the withdrawal of fluid from the tissues. This produces haemodilution and repeated estimations of the haemo-globin show a fall which varies with the amount of blood lost.

ii. Packed-cell volume (P.C.V., haematocrit). This value also falls with haemodilution and by comparing it with the fall in haemoglobin the real degree of anaemia can be assessed. In dehydration states or when plasma has been lost, e.g., burns, the P.C.V. is increased but there is no decrease in haemoglobin or the number of red cells present.

iii. Central venous pressure (see p. 100).

iv. Group and cross-match blood.

v. Measurement of the urinary output. This is reduced and may be nil when the blood-loss is severe.

TREATMENT

i. Restore blood-volume.

ii. Prevent further blood-loss.

In conditions where massive blood-loss occurs, e.g., ruptured aortic aneurysm, ruptured spleen, and ruptured ectopic gestation, prevention of further blood-loss takes priority over the restoration of blood-volume. It must also be remembered that an operation will result in further blood-loss and the induction of a general anaesthetic abolishes protective vasoconstrictor reflexes and may cause a serious fall in the blood-pressure. The clinician must be prepared for these effects.

HAEMATEMESIS AND MELAENA

CAUSES

Chronic peptic ulceration	65 per cent
Acute peptic ulceration	30 per cent
Oesophageal varices	
Cancer of the stomach	
Peptic ulcer in a Meckel's diverticulum	
Purpura	3 per cent
Haemophilia	
Pernicious and other anaemias	

CHRONIC PEPTIC ULCERATION

The bleeding usually occurs from a vessel in the posterior wall of the organ and occurs five times more often in the duodenum than in the stomach. Often a large haemorrhage is preceded by two or three smaller ones. This is particularly common in elderly patients whose atherosclerotic vessels remain open and are therefore more difficult to seal with clot.

SYMPTOMS AND SIGNS

Apart from haematemesis, melaena, and the signs of acute blood-loss there is often a past history of indigestion.

INVESTIGATIONS

i. As above for acute blood-loss.

ii. Barium or Gastrografin meal as soon as the condition of the patient permits it.

iii. Gastroscopy is playing a more important role in diagnosis in centres where it is available as a service.

TREATMENT

a. Conservative Treatment

i. The patient is laid flat and kept warm.

ii. Raise the foot of the bed.

iii. Sedation. Morphine is given intravenously or intramuscularly during the initial period as it also relieves the patient's anxiety. Other sedatives such as phenobarbitone can be used later.

iv. Replacement of the blood-volume if a moderate or severe loss has occurred.

v. No smoking.

vi. A milk drip through a nasogastric tube is favoured by some clinicians.

vii. Carbenoxolone can be given when the patient is able to take oral medication.

Progress during conservative treatment is assessed by repeating the investigations for blood-loss and by measuring the pulse-rate every $\frac{1}{4}$–$\frac{1}{2}$ hour and the blood-pressure every $\frac{1}{2}$ hour.

b. Surgical Treatment

Surgery is indicated when conservative treatment has failed or the patient is too ill to risk any delay in definitive treatment. Factors which influence the surgeon to favour operative treatment include a long history of peptic ulceration and evidence of generalized atherosclerosis.

ACUTE PEPTIC ULCERATION

It is often difficult to differentiate between this condition and chronic peptic ulceration. It may be due to drugs which either irritate the gastric mucosa, e.g., aspirin and phenylbutazone, or alter the defence mechanisms of the stomach, e.g., steroids. Other causes of acute peptic ulceration include hiatus hernia and tearing of the mucosa at the lower end of the oesophagus by violent vomiting

(Mallory–Weiss syndrome). The investigation and treatment of this condition are the same as for chronic peptic ulceration and the majority of patients settle with a conservative régime.

OESOPHAGEAL VARICES

Obstruction of the portal venous blood-flow by liver disease, etc., causes an increase in the portal venous pressure which the body attempts to reduce by opening up collaterals between the portal and systemic venous systems. This produces varices at the lower end of the oesophagus and around the fundus of the stomach which can bleed if traumatized by food, etc. However, it must also be remembered that patients with cirrhosis have an increased risk of developing gastric and duodenal ulcers. The mortality due to bleeding varices is high particularly in the presence of ascites, encephalopathy and cirrhosis.

SYMPTOMS

As well as the haematemesis and symptoms of acute blood-loss the patient gives a past history of liver disease.

SIGNS

  i. Of acute blood-loss.
 ii. Splenomegaly.
iii. Skin signs:
  a. Spider naevi.
  b. Palmar erythema.
  c. Purpura.
 iv. Ascites.
  v. Small testes, gynaecomazia, and loss of body hair.
 vi. Caput medusae at the umbilicus.

INVESTIGATIONS

  i. As for acute blood-loss.
 ii. Fibreoptic oesophagogastroscopy.

iii. Barium swallow and meal.

iv. Liver function tests and prothrombin estimation.

TREATMENT

The initial treatment is conservative and allows time to prepare the patient for definitive or palliative surgical procedures.

i. Measures used for the conservative management of chronic peptic ulceration with bleeding. Blood used to replace blood loss should be fresh and certainly not more than 48 hours old, as stored blood is low in platelets and factor V and high in potassium and ammonia. Patients with impaired liver function metabolize citrate poorly so calcium gluconate (10 ml. of 10 per cent solution) should be given with each litre of blood. Following massive blood transfusion, and in patients with deteriorating hepatic function, infusions of fresh frozen plasma and platelet-rich concentrates may be required to control haemorrhage.

ii. Phytomenadione (vitamin K) 10 mg. intravenously and 10 mg. intramuscularly.

iii. Obstetric pituitrin lowers the portal venous pressure by causing constriction of the splanchnic arterioles. The dose is 20 units in 200 ml. of normal saline given intravenously over 20 minutes. Abdominal colic, evacuation of bowels and facial pallor are the usual side effects. If they do not occur it is probable that the pituitrin is inactive and a new pack should be tried. Further doses may be required every 2 hours but the efficacy diminishes with continued use.

iv. Sengstaken tube (*Fig.* 1). This controls the haemorrhage by pressure on the bleeding varices by a balloon. The patient may be sedated with diazepam. With the head of the bed elevated the tube is passed via the mouth and when the gastric balloon is in the stomach it is inflated with 80–100 ml. of air. The tube is pulled back until the balloon impinges on the cardia and the stomach is then aspirated regularly. The oesophageal balloon is inflated with 100–200 ml. of air so that it presses on the varices and controls bleeding. It is then strapped to the patient for continuous traction. Use of these tubes is limited because:

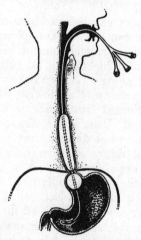

Fig. 1.—The Sengstaken tri-lumen tube and balloon.

a. The pressure may produce oesophageal ulceration or rupture if left in place for more than 72 hours.

b. Saliva collects above the balloon and has to be aspirated regularly to prevent it entering the lungs.

c. Renewed haemorrhage can occur when the tube is removed.

v. Prevention of hepatic encephalopathy which is frequently precipitated by the breakdown of blood in the bowel.

a. Correct electrolyte problems especially hypokalaemia and hypoglycaemia.

b. Magnesium sulphate enemas to clear blood from the colon.

c. Neomycin to sterilize the bowel.

vi. Surgery. This is aimed at either reducing the portal venous pressure or disconnecting the portosystemic anastomoses at the lower end of the oesophagus.

TRAUMATIC HAEMOPERITONEUM

Trauma to the abdomen produced by a crush injury or a penetrating lesion can damage the spleen, liver, mesentery, or any of the many abdominal blood-vessels and cause intraperitoneal bleeding. The patients either die quickly from profuse haemorrhage and associated injuries or come to the attention of a clinician who has to make full use of the limited time available to diagnose and carry out treatment. Usually the diagnosis of traumatic haemoperitoneum is not difficult, but as the full extent of the abdominal injury is never fully known until a laparotomy has been performed it is advisable to be prepared to find the worst at operation. A small number of patients have a delayed bleed following trauma. In these cases clot or omentum seals off the bleeding vessel temporarily or a subcapsular haematoma forms which ruptures through the capsule after 24 hours or more.

SYMPTOMS

i. Symptoms of acute blood-loss.

ii. Variable abdominal pain which is usually over the area of injury. It is made worse by the presence of fractured ribs and transverse processes.

iii. Shoulder-tip pain which is not made worse by movement.

SIGNS

i. Variable tenderness usually over the injured area.

ii. If shoulder-tip pain is not present then raising the foot of the bed should produce it as the blood collects against the inferior surface of the diaphragm.

iii. Hyperaesthesia over the shoulder tips.

iv. Abdominal rigidity (50 per cent of patients).

v. Bowel-sounds are present initially but disappear after 3–4 hours.

vi. Shifting dullness in the flanks.

vii. Tenderness on rectal examination and a soft swelling due to blood can often be felt in the rectovesical pouch.

INVESTIGATIONS

i. As for acute blood-loss.

ii. Group and cross-match 4–6 units of blood urgently.

iii. X-ray chest and abdomen if the diagnosis is not obvious after the examination. The X-rays may show:

a. Fractures of the ribs or transverse processes.

b. Loss of the splenic outline.

c. Loss of the psoas shadow on the affected side.

d. Indentation of the stomach air-bubble.

TREATMENT

This is the same as for any acute blood-loss with a laparotomy carried out as soon as possible to find and treat the source of the bleeding.

RUPTURED ECTOPIC PREGNANCY

When an ectopic pregnancy occurs the fertilized ovum may become implanted at any point along the Fallopian tube although the majority settle in its ampulla. The developing trophoblast erodes into the wall of the tube and opens up blood-vessels. When it implants in the isthmus of the tube rupture through its wall can occur so that blood escapes into the peritoneal cavity. The static, or if anything, rising death rate in this country supports the view that the incidence of ectopic pregnancy may be increasing and this has been linked with the use of intrauterine contraceptive devices and possibly progesterone-only contraceptives. These also effect the mode of presentation and may make diagnosis difficult. The amount of blood lost varies considerably and the symptoms and signs produced vary accordingly.

SYMPTOMS

   i. Symptoms of acute blood-loss.

   ii. Amenorrhoea which may vary from a few days to a few weeks over the date of the expected period.

   iii. Abdominal pain of sudden onset usually in the hypogastrium or localized to one or other iliac fossa.

   iv. Vomiting.

   v. Slight vaginal bleeding.

   vi. Fainting or feeling faint.

   vii. Shoulder-tip pain which can be produced by raising the foot of the bed.

SIGNS

   i. Signs of acute blood-loss.

   ii. Generalized abdominal tenderness with little guarding.

   iii. Normal or slightly subnormal temperature.

   iv. Pelvic examination reveals an ill-defined swelling in the pouch of Douglas due to the presence of blood.

   v. Soft cervix and acute tenderness on moving the cervix. Many gynaecologists argue that a vaginal examination should not be carried out when an ectopic pregnancy is suspected in case profuse intraperitoneal bleeding is provoked.

INVESTIGATIONS

   i. As for acute blood-loss.

   ii. Group and cross-match 4 units of blood.

DIFFERENTIAL DIAGNOSIS

This is usually not difficult, but any condition causing low abdominal pain must be considered. As well as general surgical causes these include an incomplete abortion, pelvic inflammatory disease, menstrual irregularities, dysmenorrhoea or mid cycle pain and a bleeding lutein cyst. A hydatidiform mole with vaginal bleeding may also be confused with ectopic pregnancy.

TREATMENT

i. A blood transfusion must be set up immediately and the patient treated for acute blood-loss.

ii. Surgery to remove the affected Fallopian tube.

RUPTURED ABDOMINAL ANEURYSM

An abdominal aneurysm is a dilatation of the aorta caused by a weakening of its wall by the degenerative changes of atherosclerosis. Often the first evidence of the presence of an aneurysm is leakage and once this occurs fatal frank rupture is near. As 90 per cent are situated below the level of the renal arteries they are amenable to surgery which offers some hope of cure even though emergency surgery has a mortality of between 50 and 80 per cent.

SYMPTOMS

i. Continuous abdominal and/or back pain usually in the left loin.

ii. Past history of vascular insufficiency, e.g., intermittent claudication, coronary thrombosis, or cerebrovascular accident.

SIGNS

i. Signs of blood-loss. Shock is not always present but is an ominous prognostic sign when it occurs.

ii. Abdominal mass. This is usually found in the left flank and is occasionally pulsatile.

iii. Femoral pulses may be absent.

INVESTIGATIONS

i. X-ray abdomen. This usually demonstrates a curved line of calcification in the wall of the aneurysm or a retroperitoneal mass. The best demonstration is found with a lateral view.

ii. Group and cross-match at least 8 units of blood if definitive surgery is planned.

DIFFERENTIAL DIAGNOSIS

Although the diagnosis is obvious in the majority of cases, a ruptured abdominal aortic aneurysm can masquerade as sigmoid diverticulitis, ureteric colic, and a perforated peptic ulcer. Other frequent misdiagnoses are coronary thrombosis and dissecting aneurysm.

TREATMENT

i. Replacement of blood-loss. Two drips with blood are set up and group O-negative blood given until correctly grouped blood is available. The patient must not be transfused too vigorously as this will merely raise the blood-pressure and cause further leakage from the aneurysm.

ii. Stop the bleeding. Surgery offers the only chance of cure but the poor results reported from the larger centres have caused surgeons to abandon treatment in certain circumstances. These include advanced age, a past history of coronary thrombosis or cerebrovascular accident, and the presence of severe shock.

Chapter 3

Patients presenting
with an abdominal lump

HAEMATOMA OF THE RECTUS MUSCLE

This is caused by tearing of the inferior epigastric blood-vessels and usually occurs in the rectus sheath below the linea semilunaris. Here the posterior rectus sheath is absent and the haematoma is able to expand and irritate the peritoneum, producing pain with rigidity. It may even rupture through the peritoneum into the peritoneal cavity. In these ways it is able to mimic an intraperitoneal lesion. The blood diffuses slowly through the adjacent tissues tearing the surrounding muscle-fibres and as a late sign produces bruising over the rectus sheath and sometimes in the flank as well. The amount of blood lost is variable but it can be severe and in a few cases it has proved fatal. It is claimed that many factors predispose to this condition. These include debilitating disease, senility, pregnancy, anticoagulant therapy, athletic exertion, and arterial disease.

SYMPTOMS

Soreness and later pain over the lower part of the rectus sheath. It often follows a bout of coughing or excessive muscular exertion.

SIGNS

i. A tender lump in relation to the rectus sheath. The lump does not cross the midline and can be shown to be in the abdominal wall by making the patient tense his abdominal muscles. Although this latter procedure is very painful it is a sure way of excluding any differential diagnosis which may be considered.

ii. Bruising over the lump or in the flank is a very late sign.

TREATMENT

There is very little place for a non-operative form of treatment as bleeding may continue so that a massive loss occurs. Also there is a hypothetical risk of infection occurring in the haematoma and last but not least it is often difficult to be sure of the diagnosis.

Once the blood-loss has been corrected the clot should be evacuated and the inferior epigastric vessels tied off in the rectus sheath.

IRREDUCIBLE HERNIAE

Herniae present as surgical emergencies when the contents of the sac will not return to the abdominal cavity. If there are no other complications they are simply termed *irreducible* and usually contain omentum only. The commonest obstructing factor is a tight neck to the sac but adhesions in the sac and narrowness of the hernial canal may also play a part. *Obstructed* herniae are ones in which the intestine trapped in the sac is obstructed with no interference to its blood-supply; and a *strangulated* hernia is one in which the blood-supply of the bowel is impaired producing ischaemia. It is difficult, or even impossible, to be certain that a hernia is merely obstructed and not strangulated as well. It is therefore advisable to assume that all irreducible herniae are strangulated and treat accordingly. In the case of femoral herniae this assumption is borne out more often than not.

INCIDENCE OF IRREDUCIBLE HERNIAE

Inguinal	47 per cent
Femoral	42 per cent
Para-umbilical ⎫	
Umbilical ⎬	8 per cent
Epigastric ⎭	
Incisional	3 per cent

SYMPTOMS

i. Lump. Over the appropriate hernial site.

ii. Pain. This may be the steady pain of ischaemia or the colicky pain of intestinal obstruction, although both can be present at the same time.

iii. Vomiting. Either obstructive vomiting with the nature of the vomit depending on the level of the obstruction or the reflex retching of ischaemia.

iv. Past history of hernia. This is often missing.

SIGNS

i. Absence of cough impulse over the lump.

ii. Tenderness when the contents are ischaemic.

iii. Peristalsis when obstruction is present. This may be seen either in the abdomen or the hernial sac.

INVESTIGATIONS

Many of the patients are elderly or obese and to assess their general state prior to anaesthesia a chest X-ray and E.C.G. are useful.

i. Haemoglobin and packed-cell volume.

ii. Serum electrolytes and urea if obstructive vomiting is present.

iii. Group and cross-match 2 units of blood if resection of bowel is anticipated.

Only femoral herniae may present a diagnostic problem. Firstly, when only a part of the circumference of the intestine is trapped in the sac (Richter's hernia) there may be no obvious lump. Secondly, an inflamed lymph-node over the femoral ring may simulate a femoral hernia. When this is suspected the area of lymphatic drainage should be examined for a focus of infection, i.e., lower limbs, perineum, anus, and lower abdominal wall.

TREATMENT

Manual reduction (taxis) may be attempted if the lump is not tender and has been present for less than 4 hours. No force should be used and if the manœuvre is successful an operation can be carried out at a more convenient time. If the lump is tender or has been present for more than 4 hours taxis must not be attempted as there is a danger of returning non-viable bowel to the peritoneal cavity. An operation is therefore mandatory and if the patient is considered not fit for a general anaesthetic then local anaesthesia must be used.

    i. Nasogastric aspiration.

    ii. Intravenous fluids.

    iii. Analgesics.

    iv. Antibiotics, as the fluid in the hernial sac is often teeming with bacteria.

    v. Operation.

PELVIC ABSCESS

This condition, considered here as a definite diagnosis, is often only made when a mass is found on rectal examination. This mass is a collection of purulent material which if it has not been formed in the pelvis has found its way there by gravity. At first it may produce no symptoms but it soon increases in size and may eventually be felt above the pubis. In its position the abscess lies in contact with the bladder, loops of small intestine, and the rectum and by irritating these structures produces a variety of symptoms. The patient usually presents because of these symptoms which include frequency, dysuria, intestinal obstruction or ileus, and a mucous diarrhoea. The majority of pelvic abscesses result from acute appendicitis, salpingitis, or diverticulitis. The underlying conditions may not have produced significant symptoms and signs and direct questioning is often required to elicit their history.

SYMPTOMS

i. Diarrhoea and the passage of mucus in the stools.
ii. Dysuria and urinary frequency.
iii. Intestinal obstruction or ileus.
iv. Past history of recent abdominal disturbance.

SIGNS

Rectal examination. A bulge is felt in the anterior rectal wall which, when the abscess is ripe, feels cystic. A large full bladder can be mistaken for a pelvic abscess and it is important to check the finding after the patient has voided urine.

TREATMENT

Untreated, many of these abscesses burst into the rectum and the patient makes a rapid recovery. However, the majority of cases benefit by an operation deliberately to drain the abscess once pus has formed. The presence of pus can be confirmed by aspirating the mass with a lumbar-puncture needle. Drainage can then be carried out either into the rectum or posterior fornix of the vagina.

The use of antibiotics in this condition is open to debate. On the one hand, they may reduce the constitutional disturbance caused by the condition but, on the other hand, they can slow down the actual formation of the abscess.

Chapter 4

Genito-urinary emergencies

ACUTE RETENTION OF URINE

Acute retention of urine is one of the commonest surgical emergencies encountered in the elderly male. The majority of cases are the result of benign prostatic enlargement, but other causes to be considered include prostatic carcinoma, urethral stricture, blood-clot in the bladder, acute urethritis, and phimosis or meatal stenosis. Acute retention of urine in the female is uncommon but can occur when a retroverted pregnant uterus or gynaecological mass becomes impacted in the pelvis; with urological causes such as urethral calculus, stricture or abscess, and with lesions of the spinal cord. However, the definitive treatment of these rare conditions will not be considered here.

Perhaps the commonest time acute retention of urine is met with in general surgical patients is during the immediate postoperative period when patients, especially if elderly, tend to be immobilized. The operations particularly incriminated include haemorrhoidectomy, laminectomy, abdominoperineal resection, and other pelvic operations. As would be expected the condition occurs most frequently when a patient with a past history of urinary symptoms has been given too much sedation.

ACUTE RETENTION OF URINE IN THE ELDERLY MALE PATIENT

SYMPTOMS

i. *Inability to pass any urine.* This must be differentiated from the uncontrollable persistent dribbling of chronic retention of urine with overflow which requires a different type of treatment.

ii. Past history of prostatism with hesitancy, poor stream, terminal dribbling, and nocturia.

iii. Pain is uncommon as the acute episode usually follows a chronic history.

iv. If the retention is due to a neoplastic prostate symptoms of secondary bony involvement may be found, e.g., back pain.

SIGNS

i. *Distension of the bladder*, which can be palpated or the outline percussed.

ii. *Enlargement of the prostate*, felt on rectal examination.

iii. Pin-hole external urinary meatus.

iv. Thickening along the penile urethra indicating a stricture or calculus.

v. Urethral discharge.

vi. The central nervous system must be examined, particularly the pupil reactions, knee-jerks, and cutaneous sensation in the perineum. This examination will exclude tabes dorsalis and the often-missed lesions of the spinal cord.

INVESTIGATIONS

i. Haemoglobin.

ii. Serum electrolytes and urea.

iii. Urine examination.

iv. Chest X-ray and E.C.G. examinations as the majority of patients are elderly.

v. Excretion urography (I.V.P.). Although this investigation is often omitted it is useful as not only does it give valuable information about the state of the urinary tract but bony secondaries from a carcinoma of the prostate may be seen in the spine and pelvis on the preliminary film.

vi. Cysto-urethrography if a urethral stricture is suspected.

TREATMENT

i. Catheterization (*see* p. 105). Decompression of the bladder should be carried out slowly in patients with a history of chronic retention and those with a high blood-urea. Sudden decompression in these patients can lead to severe haemorrhage from the submucosal blood-vessels.

ii. Surgery. The underlying condition is dealt with at a convenient time.

POSTOPERATIVE URINARY RETENTION

In the majority of cases no definite mechanical cause can be found although patients with some slight degree of urethral obstruction are more prone to this problem.

TREATMENT

i. Whenever possible the patient should be encouraged to sit on a commode. Lying flat in bed and trying to use a urine bottle is a potent inhibitor of micturition.

ii. Analgesics will lessen abdominal discomfort and allow adequate use of the abdominal muscles during voiding.

iii. After perineal operations spasm of the perineal muscles can be relieved by lying in a bath of warm water. The patient often finds great relief by actually voiding while bathing.

When these general methods fail the patient must be catheterized and the catheter left in place until he is fully ambulant. Then there is usually no further trouble with micturition.

TORSION OF THE TESTIS

This occurs when an abnormally mobile testis twists around its spermatic cord or, more rarely, its mesorchium.

This mobility may be due to anteversion of the testis or a high investment of the tunica vaginalis on the cord so that the testis hangs in the scrotum like a clapper in a bell. It is uncommon for the testis to be separated from the epididymis by a long mesorchium around which it is able to twist. It must be remembered that any precipitating factor present in one side of the scrotum is usually found on the other side as well. The possibility of a second torsion is therefore always present and treatment should be carried out to prevent it occurring.

The twisting movement is due to contractions of the cremaster muscle which takes its origin from the internal oblique muscle and hangs as thin loops of muscle-fibres along the spermatic cord. Any movement producing a contraction of the anterior abdominal muscles will also cause a contraction of the cremaster fibres which can initiate twisting of the spermatic cord and torsion. When the condition is untreated the testis is deprived of its blood-supply and infarction occurs within a few hours.

SYMPTOMS

    i. *Pain in the scrotum.* This is usually sudden and severe but it can present during the initial stages as a dull ache in the loin or hypogastrium.

    ii. Vomiting.

SIGNS

    i. *Tender enlarged testis,* felt separate from the cord.

    ii. *Twists can be felt along the spermatic cord.*

    iii. The affected testis lies higher than its partner.

    iv. Flexion of the leg on the affected side.

    v. Redness of the scrotal skin is a late sign and occurs after about 6 hours.

    vi. No pyrexia initially but the temperature may rise after 6 hours.

vii. Elevation and support of the scrotum does not relieve the pain.

INVESTIGATIONS

i. White blood-count is normal.

ii. Urine is sterile.

DIFFERENTIAL DIAGNOSIS

i. Acute epididymo-orchitis.

ii. Torsion of an appendage of the epididymis.

iii. A small irreducible inguinal hernia compressing the spermatic cord.

Torsion of the testis is by far the commonest cause of a painful enlarged testicle under the age of 25 years and in this age-group it is advisable to assume a diagnosis of torsion for all cases and treat as such.

TREATMENT

i. Manipulative reduction. In early cases where the twists of the cord can be felt easily it is a simple procedure to untwist the torsion. No anaesthetic is required. The testis usually twists forwards and away from the midline so reduction is carried out by gently turning the testis medially and backwards. When successful the spermatic cord returns to its normal length and shape and the patient experiences an immediate relief of pain. However, bilateral orchiopexy must be carried out at the earliest convenient time to prevent further torsions.

ii. Surgery. Orchiopexy or orchidectomy on the affected side. The 'normal' testis should also be explored and fixed at the same time because the precipitating factors that allow torsion are usually bilateral.

ACUTE EPIDIDYMO-ORCHITIS

This is an inflammation of the testis and epididymis resulting from bacterial or chemical contamination.

Bacteria reach the part from the urethra during urethral surgery or instrumentation and with gonococcal infection, but in a few cases the organism is blood-borne, e.g., mumps virus. *Escherichia coli* is by far the commonest causative organism but many others have been incriminated including staphylococci and streptococci. Acute epididymo-orchitis has also been described as a result of the passage of sterile urine along the vas deferens during micturition when the external urethral sphincter remains closed for a fractional period after the internal sphincter has opened.

SYMPTOMS

　i. *Painful, swollen epididymis and/or testicle*.

　ii. Past history of urethral surgery, instrumentation, or gonococcal infection with a urethral discharge.

　iii. Recent history of mumps or contact with mumps.

　iv. Dysuria.

　v. Malaise.

　vi. Rigors.

SIGNS

　i. *Pyrexia*.

　ii. Swollen tender scrotal contents with enlargement of the epididymis easy to feel.

　iii. Small lax hydrocele.

　iv. Elevation and support of the scrotum relieves the pain.

　v. Tenderness over the prostate or seminal vesicles on rectal examination. This must be carried out cautiously to reduce the chance of spreading the infection.

INVESTIGATIONS

　i. White blood-count shows a leucocytosis.

　ii. Microscopic examination of a mid-stream specimen of urine reveals white blood-cells and the offending organisms may be seen. The urine must be cultured.

iii. A two-glass test gives a rough guide to the site of infection. The patient is requested to pass the initial portion of the urinary stream into a collecting glass and the remainder into a second glass. When the prostate is the seat of infection only the first glass is turbid or contains debris. If both glasses are contaminated it is very probable that the infection is in the bladder.

TREATMENT

i. Bed-rest, until the acute symptoms have settled.

ii. Elevation and support of the scrotum using a nest of cotton-wool.

iii. Analgesics, e.g., pethidine.

iv. Antibiotics, e.g., ampicillin or tetracycline. Streptomycin is to be avoided until urinary tuberculosis has been completely excluded from the diagnosis.

v. High fluid intake.

vi. Surgery. Drainage of the scrotum is required when pus has formed. In cases of viral orchitis some surgeons suggest decompression of the testis by incising the tunica vaginalis. This eases the pain and may also prevent destruction of the cells concerned with spermatogenesis.

INJURY TO THE KIDNEY

The normal kidney lies in a well-protected position and a significant force is required to damage it. The commonest forces capable of injuring the kidney are a direct kick during a game of football and severe crushing injuries. When it results from a crushing accident about one-third of cases have other organs damaged and a mixture of symptoms and signs are found which may be difficult to interpret.

When a kidney is injured by relatively minor trauma the kidney is often abnormal and therefore more susceptible to damage. The degree of damage sustained by the kidney will vary from minor lacerations of the capsule and cortex to severe injury with total disruption of the kidney substance and tearing of the blood-vessels in the renal pedicle.

Damage to the renal cortex produces haematuria and when the capsule is torn a retroperitoneal haematoma is formed which may be palpable as an abdominal mass. In young children and very thin people the covering peritoneum is often torn as the perinephric fat is ill developed. This allows a mixture of urine and blood to enter the peritoneal cavity and produce symptoms and signs of peritoneal irritation.

SYMPTOMS

i. *Haematuria.* The amount of blood in the urine varies with the degree of injury. It need not occur immediately after the accident but may be delayed for up to 3 weeks after the injury.

ii. Ureteric colic as clots of blood pass down the ureter.

SIGNS

i. Of acute blood-loss.

ii. Flattening of the waist contour on the affected side. This is best seen from the front of the patient.

iii. Tenderness and rigidity over the affected side.

iv. A palpable mass (retroperitoneal haematoma) in the loin or a dullness on percussion which does not shift.

v. Meteorism as the bowel over the injured kidney distends because of the ileus.

INVESTIGATIONS

i. Haemoglobin and packed-cell volume.

ii. Serum electrolytes and urea.

These furnish base-line estimations and give a rough assessment of the blood-loss.

iii. Group and cross-match 4 units of blood.

iv. Urine examination. Every specimen of urine passed by the patient must be recorded and placed next to the previous specimen. The clinician can then note at a glance any increase or decrease in haematuria during the patient's recovery. During an uneventful recovery the urine should be examined and cultured for bacteria every 3 or 4 days.

v. X-rays.

a. Preliminary abdominal film. This may show any combination of the following signs:

1. Slight protective scoliosis concave to the affected side.

2. Loss of psoas shadow.

3. Loss of kidney contour.

4. Fractures of the ribs or transverse processes.

5. Gaseous distension of the bowel over the affected kidney (meteorism).

b. Excretion urography, preferably by a high dose infusion technique, must be carried out as soon as possible to check that the uninvolved kidney is normal and to assess the amount of damage to the affected kidney. The urographic findings may show:

1. Irregularity or disruption of the calices.

2. Leakage of the contrast medium outside the renal contour.

3. Displacement of the kidney and ureter by haematoma.

4. Non-function on the affected side.

Retrograde pyelography should not be carried out as it increases the risk of infection.

TREATMENT

Well over three-quarters of the patients make a full recovery with non-operative treatment and although the excretion urogram may not always return to normal residual sequelae such as hypertension are uncommon.

The progress and recovery during treatment can be assessed clinically and with serial urographic studies.

Conservative Treatment

i. Bed-rest, until macroscopic haematuria has been absent for 1 week.

ii. Analgesics, e.g., pethidine.

iii. Broad-spectrum antibiotics, as the traumatised kidney and perirenal haematoma are highly susceptible to infection.

iv. High fluid intake until macroscopic haematuria has resolved.

v. The pulse-rate and blood-pressure must be estimated every $\frac{1}{2}$ hour and hourly respectively during the first 24 hours and then according to the progress of the patient.

vi. As for acute blood-loss.

The indications for abandoning conservative management in favour of surgery during the initial stages are continuing deterioration as judged by unabating haematuria or an increasing loin haematoma with signs of circulatory shock.

Exploration at a later date may be considered to treat a pre-existing pelvic hydronephrosis, a perinephric abscess, an obstructing haematoma, or when partial or total loss of function occurs after an initial recovery.

INTRAPERITONEAL RUPTURE OF THE BLADDER

This results from trauma to a full bladder. There is an increase in the intravesical pressure which tears a large rent in the bladder wall and allows urine to escape into the peritoneal cavity. Classically the patient fails to pass urine after the accident and develops an ileus with increase in abdominal girth. However, the diagnosis is rarely obvious when the patient is first seen in hospital and may not be made until an exploratory laparotomy is carried out or peritonitis occurs. Treatment is closure of the rent leaving an indwelling catheter in place until healing has taken place.

EXTRAPERITONEAL RUPTURE OF THE BLADDER AND RUPTURE OF THE POSTERIOR (MEMBRANOUS) URETHRA

These conditions are considered together as they are similar in presentation. They complicate 10 per cent of fractured pelvices and occur together in one-fifth of such cases. Extravasation of urine occurs but this should not cause too much concern as urine in the tissue of the pelvis and thigh is relatively harmless for up to 36 hours. Extraperitoneal tears of the bladder are small and some urine remains in the bladder. Ninety per cent of ruptures of the posterior urethra are partial and when correctly treated the risk of subsequent troublesome urethral stricture is small. Further injury to the urethra can be prevented by not passing a urethral catheter as this may cause further tearing or introduce infection. The diagnosis should be made on clinical grounds.

SYMPTOMS
  i. Of fractured pelvis and associated shock or intra-abdominal injuries.
  ii. Has not passed urine since the accident.

SIGNS
  i. Tenderness in the hypogastrium.
  ii. Swelling in the lower abdomen usually extending to one or other side. In cases of ruptured urethra the bladder may be identified as a separate swelling.
  iii. Rising pulse-rate.
  iv. Blood at the external urethral meatus, but this is often absent.

v. Rectal examination is usually difficult because of tenderness. If the prostate cannot be felt in its normal position, or if there is a doughy sensation due to extravasated urine and blood, then there is a complete intrapelvic rupture of the urethra.

TREATMENT

i. Ask the patient not to pass urine.

ii. Broad-spectrum antibiotics.

For extraperitoneal rupture of the bladder the bladder is drained with a suprapubic catheter for 2 to 3 weeks until cystoscopy and panendoscopy confirm that the tear has healed. Partial ruptures of the posterior urethra are treated the same way with urethrography on the 10th day to check healing. Complete tears require skilled management and surgery to approximate the two cut ends of the urethra over a splint. Even then a urethral stricture is almost inevitable.

RUPTURE OF THE ANTERIOR (BULBOUS) URETHRA

This uncommon injury is caused by direct trauma to the perineum or falling astride an object so that the urethra is squashed against the pubic ramus. The pelvis is usually intact.

SIGNS

i. Retention of urine and a full bladder.

ii. Urethral haemorrhage.

iii. Perineal haematoma.

If there is doubt about the diagnosis and the patient's general condition permits, urethrography can be carried out.

TREATMENT

i. Advise patient not to pass urine.

ii. Broad-spectrum antibiotics.

ii. Analgesics.

iv. Catheter drainage of the bladder for a few days if the rupture is partial but complete ruptures require skilled surgery to drain the bladder and at a later date dilatation of the resulting stricture or urethroplasty may be required.

Chapter 5

Paediatric emergencies

INTESTINAL OBSTRUCTION OF THE NEWBORN

As many babies vomit during the first weeks of life it should not be considered serious unless it is persistent and copious or contains bile. Then a mechanical obstruction must be considered to be present until proved otherwise. The individual causes of intestinal obstruction in the newborn are rare but when all the causes are considered together they add up to a significant number. These causes include:

i. Atresia and stenosis: these are a discontinuity and a narrowing of the bowel respectively. They are believed to be the result of occlusion of intestinal blood-vessels during development and there are often several areas of obstruction in the same bowel.

ii. Malrotation: this occurs when the developing bowel fails to complete the process of rotation and fixation. The caecum remains high in the abdomen and the fibrous bands that fix it to the posterior abdominal wall cross the duodenum where they can cause obstruction. Also, instead of being attached to the posterior wall by a broad-based mesentery, the small intestine hangs by a narrow stalk which contains the superior mesenteric blood-vessels. Volvulus of the midgut around this stalk may occur so that its blood-supply is occluded.

iii. Meconium ileus: this is part of a genetically determined condition that affects the pancreas and mucus-secreting glands of both the alimentary and respiratory systems. The bowel becomes blocked with an abnormally thickened (inspissated) meconium. Unfortunately this is only a part of the child's problems as obstruction of the bronchi by mucus occurs and produces serious and persistent respiratory infections.

iv. Hirschsprung's disease: this condition is due to an absence of parasympathetic ganglion cells in the terminal colon and rectum. Peristaltic waves cannot pass across the affected segment and a functional obstruction results.

SYMPTOMS

i. *Vomiting*, which is usually persistent and copious even when feeds are withheld. It is rare for the obstruction to be proximal to the ampulla of Vater and bile to be absent from the vomit.

ii. Colic.

iii. Constipation.

SIGNS

i. Abdominal distension.

ii. Visible peristalsis.

iii. Hypothermia.

INVESTIGATIONS

i. Haemoglobin and P.C.V.   ⎱ To assess the degree
ii. Urea and serum electrolytes ⎰ of dehydration.

iii. *Group and cross-match* 1 unit of blood.

iv. *Plain X-ray of the abdomen and chest* (usually both can be seen on one film).

All babies swallow air during feeding and within the first few hours of birth the bowel contains enough air to show fluid levels. When mechanical obstruction is present loops of bowel will be seen becoming progressively more distended down to the level of the lesion which is obvious in the majority of cases. Below this site there is an opaque area.

Cases of meconium ileus show characteristic X-ray changes which differ from the other causes of obstruction in the neonate. Patterns of mottled meconium are obvious and the normal fluid levels in the bowel are absent as there is almost no fluid in the bowel lumen.

An X-ray of the chest may reveal a pneumonia caused by the aspiration of vomit.

DIFFERENTIAL DIAGNOSIS

i. Cerebral birth injuries. In almost all these cases there is a history of a difficult or precipitate delivery. Also the vomiting is accompanied by other signs of C.N.S. disturbance, e.g., irregular pulse and respirations, irritability, fits, and a tense fontanelle.

ii. Infections. Evidence of the infection is usually obvious, e.g., omphalitis and peritonitis, but urinary-tract infections must also be considered and looked for.

In these conditions a plain X-ray of the abdomen often shows distension of the bowel affecting its whole length equally and when peritonitis is present the loops of bowel may be seen to be separated by peritoneal fluid.

TREATMENT

i. *Nasogastric aspiration* must be started as soon as the diagnosis is tentatively made and once the stomach is emptied aspirations are repeated every 15 minutes. This reduces the serious risk of aspiration of vomit into the lungs.

ii. *Intravenous fluids.* A reliable drip which can be accelerated when required must be set up to give blood during the operation. Prompt and accurate replacement of blood-loss during surgery is mandatory. Unless there has been a serious delay in management the fluid and electrolyte disturbances are minimal, but if they are severe the correct treatment must be given.

iii. *Surgery*.

iv. Treatment of associated problems, e.g., antibiotics in meconium ileus for the respiratory problems.

INFANTILE HYPERTROPHIC PYLORIC STENOSIS

This condition of obscure aetiology occurs in approximately 5 of every 1000 births and is five times as common in males as in females. The obstruction is due to hypertrophy of the smooth circular muscle-fibres of the pylorus which is made complete by oedema of the pyloric mucosa. The symptoms usually occur in well-developed infants during the third to tenth weeks of life and the condition is uncommon after the third month.

SYMPTOMS

i. *Vomiting*. The vomit contains no bile. It starts as regurgitation but soon becomes regular, copious, and projectile.

ii. *Hunger*.

iii. Failure to gain weight or weight-loss.

iv. Constipation.

SIGNS

i. *Palpable pyloric tumour*. Felt while the child is feeding.

ii. *Visible gastric peristalsis*.

iii. Decreased urinary output.

iv. Hypothermia.

INVESTIGATIONS

i. Urea and serum electrolytes. There is a loss of fluid and electrolytes, particularly chlorides.

ii. Barium meal. This is only needed in doubtful cases and shows a narrow elongated pyloric canal.

DIFFERENTIAL DIAGNOSIS

i. Gastro-enteritis. The child usually has a fever, bile-stained vomit, anorexia, and frequent offensive stools.

ii. Feeding problems. These should be easily diagnosed on the history and examination.

TREATMENT

General Measures

i. *Rehydration.* An intravenous infusion of normal saline will replace both the fluid and electrolytes lost. Potassium replacement may be required if the baby has had symptoms for a long time. Blood or plasma is required in the severest cases when circulatory collapse has occurred.

ii. *Gastric lavage.* The stomach is washed out twice a day with normal saline.

Further treatment is usually surgical but medical treatment is sometimes preferred.

Medical Treatment

Antispasmodic drugs are used to relax the pylorus. Atropine methylnitrate (Eumydrin) 0·5–1·0 ml. of 1 in 10,000 alcoholic solution 20 minutes before each feed is usually sufficient.

Surgical Treatment

Ramstedt's operation divides the thickened circular muscle-fibres. Small feeds are started 4 hours after the operation and increased according to the response of the child.

IRREDUCIBLE INGUINAL HERNIA

This is almost always an indirect hernia through a patent processus vaginalis. The herniae may present at any time after birth when straining produces sufficient intra-abdominal pressure to push the abdominal contents into the sac. The sac usually contains small intestine as the omentum is still short and poorly developed at this age.

Irreducible inguinal herniae occur most commonly during the first year of life and in one-third of cases it is the first indication of the presence of a hernia. Strangulation of the contents is rare in childhood but can occur if the intestine becomes so firmly jammed that its blood-supply is impeded. More often the bowel becomes obstructed with the child soon developing symptoms and signs that make the diagnosis obvious.

SYMPTOMS AND SIGNS

i. *Swelling* of variable size originating at the external inguinal ring.

ii. A past history of hernia.

iii. Pain.

iv. Vomiting, usually reflex but occasionally obstructive in type.

TREATMENT

i. *Conservative Treatment*

This is the best initial treatment as 90 per cent of cases reduce themselves without requiring emergency surgery. But it must not be tried if: (1) the lump is tender, (2) there is redness or oedema of the skin over the hernia, (3) the vomit is either bile stained or faeculent.

a. Sedation, e.g., nepenthe.

b. Taxis. Either using gentle pressure with the hand or by placing the child on its back and suspending the legs from a gallows traction, e.g., Balkan beam.

If taxis is successful a herniotomy can be carried out on the next convenient list, by which time any oedema of the sac will have had time to settle. If reduction has not occurred within 3 hours then an operation is required.

ii. *Surgical Treatment*

This consists of reduction of the contents and a herniotomy. Resection of the bowel may be needed but this is very rare.

ACUTE APPENDICITIS

This is the commonest condition requiring intra-abdominal surgery in childhood and if left untreated it can run a rapid and fatal course. Most cases are readily diagnosed but the atypical ones present difficult diagnostic problems. Children over the age of 5 years present in a similar way to adults but under this age the condition is not rare and the clinical picture is somewhat different.

Acute appendicitis in young children is accompanied by an increased morbidity and mortality. This is due to delay and difficulty in diagnosis as only a third of children present within 24 hours of the onset of symptoms; and 80 per cent of children have peritonitis when they present as perforation occurs early and the omentum, being poorly developed, is unable to limit the spread of infection.

SYMPTOMS

The onset is vague and the initial symptoms are rather general.

i. *Pain.* Usually constant around the umbilicus.

ii. *Vomiting.*

iii. Constipation. This is not uncommon but the younger the child the greater is the incidence of diarrhoea.

iv. Anorexia.

v. Thirst.

vi. Irritability.

SIGNS

i. *Tenderness and guarding* often localized to the right iliac fossa.

ii. *Pyrexia.*

iii. Dry furred tongue with foetor oris.

iv. Increasing pulse-rate.

v. Abdominal distension with restricted abdominal movements.

vi. Bowel-sounds are often absent but young children can have normal bowel-sounds in the presence of peritonitis.

vii. Rectal examination is usually not helpful but may reveal either tenderness or a mass in the pelvis.

INVESTIGATIONS

i. White blood-count. This is usually elevated but it is not unknown for a child with a diffuse peritonitis to have a normal white blood-count.

ii. Urine examination. To exclude a urinary infection.

DIFFERENTIAL DIAGNOSIS

Many conditions must be considered including respiratory infection, intestinal obstruction, mesenteric lymphadenitis, pyelitis, gastro-enteritis, and infective hepatitis. It must also be remembered that acute appendicitis can occur with any of these conditions.

TREATMENT

i. *Appendicectomy.*

ii. Intravenous infusion if the child is dehydrated.

iii. Nasogastric aspiration if peritonitis and ileus are present.

iv. Antibiotics in cases with peritonitis. Ampicillin 250 mg. intramuscularly every 6 hours until the ileus has settled and then it can be given orally. The ampicillin may be given alone or in combination with streptomycin 40 mg. per kg. per day in divided doses.

INTUSSUSCEPTION

Intussusception is an invagination of one portion of the intestine into another and almost always occurs in the direction of peristalsis. The commonest types (90 per cent of cases) are the ileocaecal and ileocolic where the terminal ileum with its mesentery is drawn into the colon, and if they are left untreated gangrene results owing to compression of the blood-vessels. The morbidity and mortality of the condition are directly related to the duration of symptoms and signs.

Intussusception is the commonest cause of intestinal obstruction during the first 5 years of life and has its maximum incidence between the ages of 3 and 18 months. No single factor is responsible for this condition, but the majority of the children also have enlargement of the lymphatic patches in the terminal ileum. These may project into the lumen of the bowel and act as the apex of the intussusception as the bowel, treating them as a bolus of food, moves them along by peristalsis. This lymphatic enlargement can occur during weaning, as part of a generalized viral lymphadenitis, or with respiratory infections. Intussusception may also occur with gastro-enteritis, Henoch–Schönlein purpura, and in children possessing a Meckel's diverticulum.

SYMPTOMS

Classically the condition occurs in a healthy infant who has been developing quite normally.

i. *Colic.* The spasms make the child scream out, draw up its knees, and roll over on to its abdomen. Between pains the child lies quite still.

ii. Vomiting.

iii. Constipation or redcurrant-jelly stools after passing one or two normal stools.

SIGNS

i. *Pallor*, with each spasm of pain.

ii. Empty rectum but fresh blood or mucus is often present. Very rarely the apex of the intussusception can be felt.

iii. Tachycardia.

iv. Bowel-sounds are reduced between pains and increased during them.

v. Abdomen is soft between pains and the right iliac fossa feels empty.

vi. Palpable mass in the abdomen which is occasionally sausage-shaped.

vii. Pyrexia or a subnormal temperature.

INVESTIGATIONS

i. Urea and serum electrolytes.

ii. Group and cross-match 1 unit of blood.

iii. X-rays.

a. Plain abdomen (erect and supine) shows fluid levels in progressively dilating loops of bowel and an absence of gas shadows on the right side of the abdomen.

b. Barium enema if the diagnosis is still in doubt.

DIFFERENTIAL DIAGNOSIS

i. Volvulus. In the absence of X-ray facilities this diagnosis can be difficult but shock occurs more quickly in volvulus. The differentiation is somewhat academic as the treatment is essentially the same.

ii. Gastro-enteritis. The onset of gastro-enteritis is not so dramatic as intussusception. The colic is rarely as severe and vomiting is usually a more prominent feature. However, the clinician must beware as intussusception frequently occurs with gastro-enteritis.

TREATMENT

i. *General Preparation*

a. Intravenous infusion of normal saline to replace the fluid lost.

b. Plasma or blood if the child is shocked.

c. Broad-spectrum antibiotics, as there is a risk of septicaemia if devitalized bowel is present.

ii. *Surgery*

Usually only reduction of the intussusception with or without appendicectomy is required but, very rarely, resection of ischaemic bowel may be necessary. There is a recurrence rate of 3 per cent following surgery.

iii. *Non-surgical Treatment*

This form of treatment is only justified on the very rare occasion when surgery cannot be carried out. The intussusception is reduced by inserting saline, air, or barium into the colon via the rectum. It carries a risk of perforating the bowel wall, a high incidence of recurrence, and nearly one-quarter of the patients require operative treatment at a later date as the reduction is incomplete.

Chapter 6

Medical conditions producing an 'acute abdomen'

It has been estimated that at least one-sixth of patients admitted to hospital as surgical emergencies are actually suffering from medical conditions. Accurate diagnosis of these conditions is obviously important, as operations on patients with such commonly confused conditions as coronary thrombosis and pneumonia could end in disaster. The most frequently encountered problems occur with intrathoracic disease where upper abdominal pain and rigidity can be produced by involvement of the intercostal nerves which also supply the abdominal wall (*Table* 4). Such errors can be avoided if the surgeon is aware of the problem and examines the chests of all his patients. However, it must be remembered that acute medical and surgical conditions can occur simultaneously. Also it is not unknown for a past history of an acute medical condition such as a coronary thrombosis to cause confusion when the patient is later admitted to hospital with a similar story but this time due to a surgical condition such as a perforated peptic ulcer.

MYOCARDIAL INFARCTION

The pain produced by a myocardial infarction is sudden, severe, and not relieved by rest or vasodilator drugs. It has a wide distribution and can occur in one or more of the following regions: the sternal area, epigastrium, jaw,

Table 4. DIFFERENCES BETWEEN RIGIDITY OF THE ABDO-
MINAL MUSCLES CAUSED BY SURGICAL AND MEDICAL
CONDITIONS

SURGICAL	MEDICAL
i. The patient prefers to lie down except during spasms of colic which will cause him to move about trying to find a comfortable position	The patient prefers to sit up
ii. Usually the pain lasts longer than 6 hours	The pain is usually settling within 6 hours
iii. The rigidity persists after morphine has been given	Morphine diminishes the rigidity
iv. The rigidity persists when thoracic respiration is prevented by firm pressure on the sternum	Abdominal respiration occurs when thoracic respiration is prevented
v. When the rigidity is unilateral pressure on the opposite side of the abdomen produces pain	Contralateral pressure does not produce pain

and the arms. When the pain is atypical and confined to the epigastrium it can mimic such conditions as a perforated peptic ulcer and acute pancreatitis.

The patient with a myocardial infarction is shocked, hypotensive, and has a tachycardia. If the patient's usual blood-pressure is known it will be noted that the systolic level is greatly reduced while the diastolic reading is little altered. A mild fever and central or peripheral circulatory failure may be present. When the infarction extends to the epicardial surface a pericardial rub can be heard. Investigations are invaluable when the diagnosis is in doubt.

ELECTROCARDIOGRAPHY

The changes of myocardial infarction may take several hours to appear and they occur in the following order.

i. An elevation of the S–T segment which settles after a day or two.

ii. A pathological Q wave which is both deeper and wider than the physiological Q wave and persists indefinitely. The R deflexion is correspondingly reduced and may be absent.

iii. T-wave inversion which takes months or years to disappear.

When the epicardium is not involved S–T elevation and pathological Q waves do not occur and the diagnosis depends on the appearance of deep symmetrically inverted T waves. The leads in which changes are seen indicate the position of the infarct and the artery occluded:

a. Anteroseptal (anterior descending branch of the left coronary). Leads: V2–4; I and VL.

b. Anterolateral (left circumflex branch). Leads: V5–6; I, II, and VL.

c. Posterior (right coronary). Leads: III and VF.

Abdominal distension causing a horizontal heart can also produce Q waves and inverted T waves in leads III and VF. However, there is no S–T elevation and these changes disappear with deep inspiration.

ENZYME CHANGES

The serum glutamic oxaloacetic transaminase (S.G.O.T.) becomes raised above 40 Sigma Frankel units in 80 per cent of patients with myocardial infarction.

A leucocytosis and raised sedimentation rate are produced by the muscle necrosis after several days.

CONGESTIVE CARDIAC FAILURE

Congestive cardiac failure can produce upper abdominal pain and vomiting when the liver is rapidly distended and its capsule stretched. Other signs of cardiac failure such as distension of the neck veins, cardiac enlargement, peripheral oedema, triple rhythm or pulsus alternans, and basal crepitations are usually present. There may be a history of cardiac or chronic chest disease and symptoms of dyspnoea, cough, and recent anorexia.

PLEURITIC PAIN

Pleurisy may produce abdominal pain with guarding when the lower six thoracic nerves are irritated by a lower-lobe pneumonia or a pulmonary infarct. In these conditions the respiratory rate is increased and the respirations are shallow. Physical examination will reveal diminished chest movements and a pleural rub or signs of consolidation may be present. A chest X-ray will confirm the diagnosis.

DIABETIC KETOSIS

Impending diabetic coma may be accompanied by severe abdominal pain with guarding and vomiting. These symptoms only occur in badly controlled diabetics but can be the initial mode of presentation for an occult diabetic. Although the patient's level of consciousness varies from slight drowsiness to complete coma other symptoms and signs are always present. These include thirst, polyuria, constipation, muscle cramps, and visual disturbances. Copious vomiting may be present but unlike the vomiting of acute surgical conditions it occurs before the onset of pain. Signs of dehydration and air hunger are present and a smell of acetone can be detected on the breath.

It must be remembered that the presence of glucosuria or ketosis does not exclude an intra-abdominal condition which may be coexistent and even have precipitated the coma. Also children with repeated vomiting soon become dehydrated and produce ketosis which may confuse the diagnosis. Investigations that help to confirm the diagnosis include:

    i. The urine of all patients with abdominal pain must

be examined for sugar and when present the urine should also be tested for ketones.

ii. The blood-sugar level is raised to the range 22–44 mmol per litre (400–800 mg. per cent) but it may be higher.

iii. The plasma bicarbonate level and blood pH are low.

iv. Serum sodium and potassium levels are normal or raised.

The presence of a leucocytosis does not help as it is usual in both diabetic coma and inflammatory conditions. It may be difficult to differentiate the cause of the pain, but when the ketosis is correctly treated with insulin and glucose the symptoms due to the ketosis rapidly disappear. If the symptoms and signs do not subside then an intra-abdominal condition is present.

BORNHOLM DISEASE
(EPIDEMIC PLEURODYNIA)

This condition is caused by the Coxsackie virus B and as it usually occurs as an epidemic its diagnosis rarely presents a problem. The patient experiences a sudden pain in the abdomen or chest which is aggravated by movements and may be severe enough to produce shock. The symptoms last from 10 days to several weeks. It is usually accompanied by fever, headache, flitting muscle pains, and superficial hyperaesthesia. Other symptoms and signs of abdominal and thoracic disease are absent and no leucocytosis is present.

HERPES ZOSTER (SHINGLES)

Herpes zoster is produced by invasion of the posterior root ganglia by the varicella (chicken-pox) virus. When the lower thoracic intercostal nerves are involved the patient experiences a constant band-like pain and paraesthesia over the area of abdominal wall supplied by the nerves. Within a few days a characteristic vesicular eruption appears on the skin over the involved area. There may be a history of contact with chicken-pox or an epidemic of herpes to help to confirm the diagnosis.

ACUTE INTERMITTENT PORPHYRIA

Patients with this rare condition excrete large amounts of porphyrins in the urine and can present with colicky abdominal pain and vomiting. Porphyrins are iron-free pigments produced during haemoglobin metabolism and normally do not appear in the free state. The condition is due to a disorder of pyrrole metabolism and the diagnosis can be made by detecting porphyrin precursors in the patient's urine. The urine may be a normal colour when fresh but if acidified and allowed to stand in the light the precursors are converted to a deep red-brown porphyrin pigment. This colour change is most marked near the surface where it is in contact with air. The abnormal pigment can also be identified spectroscopically.

The symptoms are caused by smooth-muscle contraction and even when very severe there is usually a complete absence of abdominal signs. Associated neurological changes such as mental disturbances, fits, and flaccid paralysis can lead to an incorrect diagnosis of hysteria. The symptoms can be precipitated by barbiturates, sulphonamides, or pregnancy. Often a family history of the condition can be obtained.

HENOCH'S (ANAPHYLACTOID) PURPURA

This condition of obscure aetiology can occur at any age and is best described as a non-thrombocytopaenic purpura affecting the skin, mucous membranes, and joints. When the bleeding occurs into the bowel wall colicky abdominal pain, vomiting, and distension can result. The condition may also present as either intussusception or melaena.

A past or family history of allergy is often elicited and skin purpura often follows the onset of abdominal pain. Mild fever is usual and investigations will reveal a raised sedimentation rate, hypergammaglobulinaemia, and a normal platelet count.

URAEMIA

The uraemia of chronic renal failure can produce a sudden and intense vomiting similar to that found with a high intestinal obstruction. Diarrhoea or a change in bowel habit are often present. However, the patient's past history plus other signs of uraemia and the absence of the abdominal signs of intestinal obstruction will guide the clinician to the correct diagnosis.

Chapter 7

Postoperative problems

A. POSTOPERATIVE PYREXIA

The cause of a postoperative pyrexia may be difficult to determine and the clinician must systematically check for the following in each case.

a. Chest complications: these include bronchitis, bronchopneumonia, and bronchopulmonary segmental collapse. They occur most frequently in smokers, patients with chronic bronchitis or emphysema, and following operations involving the upper abdomen. In these high-risk patients therapy must be started before the operation.

PREOPERATIVE PREPARATION

i. Patients must be as ambulant as possible.

ii. Smoking must be stopped.

iii. Assisted postural coughing and deep-breathing exercises.

iv. Bronchospasm can be relieved by ephedrine tabs. 30 mg. t.d.s. (care being taken with elderly men as it can cause wakefulness and urinary retention) or an isoprenaline spray.

v. Antibiotics, e.g., ampicillin or tetracycline. A specimen of sputum must be sent for culture first.

Once infection has occurred a specimen of sputum must be sent for culture and a chest X-ray obtained.

TREATMENT

i. If a mucus plug is blocking a large bronchus or the patient is not expectorating the mucus being produced, then bronchoscopy and aspiration must be carried out.

ii. Nasogastric tubes should be removed as they interfere with coughing—with the exception of patients with a depressed cough reflex where there is a danger of inhalation of vomit.

iii. Analgesics, avoiding opiates which depress respirations, and codeine which suppresses the cough reflex. A combination of pethidine 25–50 mg. and promethazine 25 mg. given intramuscularly every 4 hours is very useful.

iv. Antibiotics.

v. Rigorous physiotherapy with postural coughing.

vi. Oxygen, if required.

b. Localized infection: this usually occurs in the wound but may be found at the operation site, in the pelvis, or, more rarely, in the subphrenic region.

c. Reaction to a blood transfusion.

d. Deep-vein thrombosis in the legs or pelvis.

e. Pulmonary embolus.

f. Urinary infection, if the patient has been catheterized during the operation or to empty the bladder for a postoperative retention. A mid-stream or catheter specimen of urine must be cultered and a suitable antibiotic given.

g. Sensitivity reaction to drugs, e.g., halothane anaesthesia.

h. Septicaemia following the administration of intravenous fluids or when the patient's resistance is low, e.g., diabetes mellitus, cirrhosis.

i. Pylephlebitis following intra-abdominal . infection may be recognized by rigors, icteric tinge, and liver enlargement.

B. WOUND DEHISCENCE

Dehiscence of an abdominal wound occurs in a small percentage of patients following laparotomy and allows intestine to escape from the peritoneal cavity. Although dehiscence tends to occur between the sixth and tenth days after operation the actual process of disruption of the wound starts in the deep layers sooner, if not immediately after the operation. In the majority of cases there is a warning pink, serous fluid discharge from the wound a day or two before the whole wound disrupts. At this stage the intestine is lying extraperitoneally and often the patient claims to have felt 'something give way' a short time earlier.

Factors which contribute to wound dehiscence include surgical misjudgement (unfortunately this is the commonest cause), infection, abdominal distension, deficiency of vitamin C or protein, and steroid therapy. Vertical incisions dehisce more often than other incisions.

The symptoms and signs of this condition are obvious but surprisingly the patient is rarely shocked or complains of pain.

TREATMENT

i. Cover the wound and exposed intestine with sterile cloths.

ii. Nasogastric aspiration.

iii. Intravenous fluids.

iv. Antibiotics, e.g., systemic ampicillin or a combination of penicillin and streptomycin.

v. Resuture the abdominal wound under general anaesthesia as soon as is possible.

The resutured wound usually heals quickly and without trouble as the healing changes have already started in the wound edges and they are able to continue once more.

C. DEEP-VEIN THROMBOSIS (D.V.T.) AND PULMONARY EMBOLISM (P.E.)

A thrombus forming in the deep veins of the lower limbs and pelvis threatens the patient with either death from a P.E. or the destruction of venous valves leading to severe post-thrombotic effects, e.g., varicose ulceration. Pulmonary embolism kills at least 2500 people in the United Kingdom every year and contributes to more than 9 per cent of all hospital deaths. It is therefore disappointing to find that vigorous research into D.V.T. and its prevention has not altered the incidence of P.E. during the past 50 years; in fact it has only revealed that D.V.T. occurs much more frequently than clinicians had previously suspected.

Over 70 per cent of patients with a P.E. give no precursory clinical evidence of D.V.T. as in the majority of cases the clot forms in the veins of the pelvis where it can become quite extensive without occluding the veins. These figures have shown how inadequate is the routine examination of the lower limbs of hospital patients in order to diagnose D.V.T. earlier and institute more effective treatment. Very rarely the embolus forms in the heart either on a healed area of infarction or as a result of atrial fibrillation.

To add to the problems of diagnosis between 30 and 50 per cent of patients with a clinical diagnosis of D.V.T. are found to have normal veins when investigated by phlebography. It is therefore essential to confirm the diagnosis in all but the most obvious cases of D.V.T. with more specific investigations before carrying out treatment which can be complicated, costly, and harmful.

The recent use of more sophisticated investigations has shown that the overall incidence of D.V.T. after major surgery on middle-aged and elderly patients is as high as 30 per cent and that thrombosis starts during the operation or very soon after it. Over 60 per cent of thromboses were detected within 2 days of operation and only 5 per cent after the first week. Factors which increase the risk of D.V.T. in a patient include:

  i. Age. D.V.T. being commoner in the elderly.

ii. Obesity.

iii. Atheromatous disease and heart failure.

iv. Immobility.

v. Oral contraceptives, particularly those with a high oestrogen content.

vi. Certain operations, e.g., splenectomy, hip replacement, and retropubic prostatectomy.

vii. Certain conditions, e.g., carcinoma of the pancreas.

When emboli formed in the systemic veins pass through the right side of the heart into the pulmonary artery they lodge either in the main trunk or in one of its branches. The effects produced are usually related to the size of the embolus, but they are not entirely the result of mechanical obstruction of the artery as even small emboli can cause death by reflex vasoconstriction of the pulmonary blood-vessels. In less than 15 per cent of fatal cases of P.E. are the emboli confined to a single lung, and when emboli in a single lung are sufficient to cause death the patients are usually over 50 years of age. In a young patient even large pulmonary emboli produce few serious cardiovascular effects if confined to one lung.

DEEP-VEIN THROMBOSIS

SYMPTOMS

i. *Pain* in the calf or along the course of the saphenous veins.

ii. Pulmonary embolism.

SIGNS

Although the affected limb should always be compared with the 'normal' limb, it must not be forgotten that the condition can be bilateral.

i. *Ankle oedema.*

ii. *Local tenderness* over the calf or along the saphenous veins.

iii. *A spike of temperature.*

iv. Dilated superficial veins.

v. Increased skin temperature of the affected limb.

vi. Pain in the calf on dorsiflexion of the foot.

Until recently clinical examination has been the only method of diagnosing a D.V.T., but investigation techniques are now being developed which it is hoped will correct this problem. These include:

i. Phlebography. Contrast medium injected into a superficial vein on the dorsum of the foot is prevented from leaving the leg by a tourniquet placed above the knee. The contrast medium enters the deep veins which are then viewed on an X-ray screen. When the tourniquet is removed the more proximal veins can be examined as the venous flow returns to normal. The presence of a thrombus can be confirmed by this examination and its exact site, size, and nature determined.

The examination takes only a short time to perform and causes little discomfort for the patient. Complications are minimal but damage to the intima of the vessel wall may occur and there is a very small risk of a thrombus being dislodged into the circulation. Unfortunately the use of phlebography is limited. There has to be a clinical indication to justify its use and it is therefore impracticable as a screening technique.

ii. Radioactive fibrinogen technique. As thrombus formed in veins uses fibrinogen from the blood, any radioactive fibrinogen injected intravenously will also be incorporated into the structure of the clot and can be detected by an oscillation counter. The fibrinogen used for this test is labelled with radioactive iodine ^{125}I which has a half-life of 60 days and can therefore be stored before use and will remain in the circulation for a reasonable period. Before it is injected into the patient the uptake of iodine by the thyroid must be blocked by potassium iodide given 24 hours before the test and daily for the following 3 weeks.

Counts are made every day over selected points in the lower limb and compared with counts over the precordial area. Increases in the count over a deep vein indicate thrombus formation.

The technique is very accurate, simple to perform, and causes no discomfort for the patient. Unfortunately it has limitations which restrict its use to research at present. These include:

α. Useless for diagnosing thrombus in the upper femoral and iliac veins. But it is noteworthy that when the radioactive test is negative, pulmonary embolism is very rare.

β. Unreliable in the presence of healing wounds of the lower limbs as these also take up fibrinogen.

γ. Inaccurate in the presence of gross oedema as the radioactive iodine diffuses into the oedema fluid.

δ. Contra-indicated in pregnancy and patients under the age of 40 years.

TREATMENT

Treatment must not be started until a definite diagnosis has been made. There is no universal method of treating D.V.T. but most schemes include the following:

a. General Measures

i. *Bed-rest,* until the acute symptoms have disappeared. The foot of the bed is elevated 10–20 cm. to encourage venous return.

ii. *Firm bandaging* with elastic bandages applied firmly from the toes to the groin compress superficial veins and encourage flow in the deep veins.

iii. Leg exercises should be performed at regular intervals. The risk of provoking a P.E. is negligible.

iv. Analgesics, e.g., aspirin or phenylbutazone, are usually sufficient.

b. Specific Drugs

i. *Anticoagulants*

α. Heparin. This inhibits various enzyme systems concerned with coagulation and in high doses may also prevent aggregation of platelets by thrombin. It is given by intravenous infusion so the dose can be adjusted by varying the rate of drip. Intramuscular injections can result in haematomas and have a less predictable anticoagulant effect.

The clotting time of the patient is estimated before treatment is started and maintained at approximately twice this control value during treatment. If bleeding does occur the effects of heparin wear off rapidly as it is metabolized speedily in the body and apart from stopping the infusion, treatment is rarely required. When further treatment is needed protamine sulphate is given by slow intravenous injection. Each 10 mg. neutralizes 500 units of heparin.

β. Oral anticoagulants. These act as substrate competitors for the vitamin K required during the synthesis of various clotting factors. They are not effective until 24–48 hours after oral administration and are given twice a day as their effect lasts for only 12–16 hours. The dose is regulated by estimations of the prothrombin time which should be kept at between one and a half and twice the control value. When treatment is complicated by bleeding the drug must be stopped and vitamin K (Phytomenadione) 10–20 mg. given intravenously. This will stop the bleeding within 12–24 hours but occasionally after severe bleeding a transfusion of fresh blood is also necessary.

The method of anticoagulating a patient varies from clinician to clinician. Usually heparin and oral anticoagulants are started in combination and the heparin stopped once the oral preparations have had time to become effective. However, there is a lot in favour of only giving a course of heparin when treating D.V.T.

ii. *Defibrinating and Fibrinolytic Agents*

α. Ancrod (Arvin) obtained from Malayan pit viper venom has a specific coagulant action on fibrinogen converting it to micro-clots which are rapidly eliminated from the circulation. When administered by an intravenous infusion or deep intramuscular injection ancrod can keep the plasma fibrinogen at a very low level and prevent extension of a thrombus. It is easy to control and bleeding is relatively uncommon but in time antibodies develop to it.

β. Streptokinase and urokinase. These substances convert plasminogen to plasmin which has a proteolytic effect on the fibrin and fibrinogen of the thrombus. They are given by slow intravenous infusion and have their greatest effect when injected directly into the thrombus particularly if it has been present for less than 96 hours.

c. Surgery

Surgical intervention is necessary when limb viability is threatened, if anticoagulants are contra-indicated, or where these measures have failed to prevent pulmonary emboli.

MASSIVE PULMONARY EMBOLISM

Massive pulmonary emboli are often rapidly fatal within a short period of time and it is unlikely that any treatment can reduce this initial high mortality. Obstruction to the pulmonary circulation is maximum at the moment of impact. From then on time lapse represents improvement during which the embolus shrinks, fragments and re-embolizes to the periphery of the lung. Patients who survive a near fatal pulmonary embolism usually improve rapidly and in 6–12 hours are out of danger and, unless further emboli reach the lungs, they have lost the signs of circulatory obstruction by 48 hours.

SYMPTOMS (sudden onset of)

i. *Severe chest pain.*

ii. *Intense dyspnoea.*
iii. *Feeling of impending death* from suffocation.
iv. Desire to defaecate.

SIGNS

i. *Hypotension.*
ii. *Engorgement of neck veins.*
iii. Peripheral cyanosis and vasoconstriction.
iv. Triple rhythm.
v. Accentuated pulmonary second sound.

PULMONARY EMBOLISM WITH PULMONARY INFARCTION

SYMPTOMS

i. *Chest pain* usually of a pleuritic type.
ii. Dyspnoea.
iii. Blood-stained sputum.

SIGNS

i. *Increased respiratory rate.*
ii. *Moderate pyrexia.*
iii. *Tachycardia.*
iv. Pallor and peripheral cyanosis.
v. Accentuated pulmonary second sound and pleural friction rub.
vi. Dilated neck veins.
vii. Sweating.
viii. Hypotension.

The symptoms and signs of P.E. can resemble a variety of conditions, e.g., myocardial infarction, spontaneous pneumothorax, pneumonia. It may also simulate an intra-abdominal catastrophe and vice versa. Before treatment is decided upon the diagnosis must be definite and the following investigations can help:

i. *White blood-count* reveals a polymorphonuclear leucocytosis.

ii. *E.C.G.* This is useful for ruling out myocardial infarction as patients with minor emboli and a few with massive emboli show no E.C.G. abnormalities. The E.C.G. should be repeated frequently if pulmonary embolism is suspected because changes may be delayed, transient or only recognized in serial records. The following changes are not specific for P.E. but any may be present:

a. Atrial fibrillation.

b. ST segment depression. This is the most frequent finding and is probably the result of associated myocardial ischaemia.

c. Enlargement of the P wave.

d. T-wave inversion, particularly in leads III, aVF, V_1, V_4, and V_5.

iii. Chest X-ray. This will help to rule out pneumonia and congestive heart failure. Although there may be no radiological changes any of the following may be present:

a. Diminished pulmonary vascular markings—usually asymmetrical. This finding occurs in about 50 per cent of patients but returns to normal within 48 hours.

b. Pleural or linear opacities (atelectasis), often bilateral.

c. Enlargement of the pulmonary artery and right ventricle. This indicates an unfavourable prognosis.

d. Pleural effusion.

e. Elevation of the diaphragm on the affected side.

iv. Central venous pressure (C.V.P.). The C.V.P. is raised when right ventricular failure occurs and a pulmonary embolus can be ruled out if there is both systemic hypotension and a low C.V.P. This procedure also makes it possible to obtain blood samples for blood–gas estimations and to deliver drugs close to the site of embolization.

v. Blood–gas analysis. Both the Po_2 and Pco_2 are reduced during an acute P.E. and a normal Po_2 rules out a P.E. Repeated estimations provide a valuable guide to oxygen therapy.

vi. Changes in serum enzymes. These have a very limited value as they take too long to estimate but they can occasionally help in differentiating a P.E. from a myocardial infarction. The changes in P.E. include elevation of serum lactic dehydrogenase and increased or normal serum bilirubin concentration with a normal glutamic oxalo-acetic transaminase (S.G.O.T.).

vii. Radio-isotope scanning using serum albumin tagged with ^{131}I and pulmonary arteriography are useful in the few centres where they are available.

TREATMENT

The majority of patients are managed by medical treatment and the cardiovascular effects produced by even large emboli are almost normal within 2 weeks because emboli tend to undergo a spontaneous regression in size. Prophylaxis is the best method of treatment and precautions should be taken for patients in the high-risk groups for developing a D.V.T. These precautions include compression of the superficial veins of the lower limbs with elastic bandages or stockings and elevation of the foot of the bed 10–20 cm. Both these measures improve the flow of blood in the deep veins. Occasionally prophylactic anticoagulant therapy may be required especially when there is a past history of D.V.T. or P.E. In such cases low doses of heparin may be given subcutaneously. 5000 units are given 2 hours before surgery and repeated every 8 hours for 7 days or until the patient is fully mobile. There is, however, an increased risk of wound haematoma.

Medical Treatment
   i. Bed-rest.

ii. Analgesics, e.g., morphine which also reduces the apprehension.

iii. Oxygen administered by face mask, nasal catheter, or tracheal intubation is an absolute 'must'. Hypoxia occurs immediately and can produce arrhythmias or myocardial and cerebral ischaemia. Arterial Po_2 should be measured at intervals to check that the oxygen supply is adequate.

iv. Antibiotics to reduce the risk of infection in the infarcted area, e.g., ampicillin or a combination of penicillin and streptomycin.

v. *Anticoagulants*. This is the primary method of treatment for the majority of patients and a continuous infusion drip of heparin is the drug of choice. As well as its anticoagulant properties heparin also has an effect on the reflex bronchoconstriction. Only heparin should be used during the acute stages and the dose regulated to maintain the clotting time at twice normal. Oral anticoagulants can be started at a later date if preferred to heparin.

vi. Fibrinolytic agents may have a part to play but at present they should be used with care.

Surgical Treatment

Pulmonary embolectomy may be indicated in the severest cases but even with an experienced surgeon the mortality is high.

D. ACUTE DILATATION OF THE STOMACH

This is a form of paralytic ileus confined to the stomach in which the stomach dilates and may reach an enormous size. It occurs suddenly and usually after abdominal operations, the application of a plaster-of-Paris jacket, or any moderate or severe trauma. It has become relatively uncommon during recent years owing to the widespread practice of using nasogastric aspiration after abdominal operations. However, clinicians must still remain aware of its possibility and make the diagnosis before vomiting occurs as this is a relatively late symptom.

SYMPTOMS

i. *Abdominal discomfort.*

ii. *Occasional hiccough.*

iii. Repeated effortless vomiting of large quantities of brownish-black fluid.

SIGNS

i. *Rising pulse.*

ii. *Scanty output of urine.*

iii. Slight fullness in the hypochondria.

iv. Succussion splash present.

v. Pallor.

vi. Hypotension.

TREATMENT

Treatment should be carried out whenever the diagnosis is suspected on clinical evidence.

i. *Nasogastric aspiration*, removing all the stomach content initially and then aspirating regularly every 15–30 minutes.

ii. *Intravenous fluids* giving normal saline to replace the volume of fluid aspirated from the stomach. Further fluid is given according to the clinical condition of the patient and the results of urea and electrolyte estimations.

iii. Blood transfusion if the blood-pressure remains low after the initial treatment.

Gastric dilatation can recur after treatment has stopped and the patient should therefore be observed carefully for a further 24–48 hours.

E. 'BACTERIAEMIC SHOCK'

This is a state of collapse caused by bacteria or their

products entering the circulation. It particularly affects patients at the extremes of life, for two-thirds of all cases occur in the first, seventh, and eighth decades. The mortality from this condition varies between 30 and 75 per cent, and during the past 25 years its incidence has increased so that it is now second only to myocardial infarction as a cause of death in hospital patients. Approximately two-thirds of the cases are the result of infection by Gram-negative bacilli and the remaining one-third produced by Gram-positive organisms.

The systemic effects are believed to be produced by endotoxins liberated from the cell wall of organisms which either are present in the blood or have access to the circulation. The endotoxins or bacteria produce their effects either by direct action on the heart muscle and blood-vessels or by an indirect action on the nervous mechanisms regulating the cardiovascular system. These cause a pooling of blood in the venous system so that venous return to the heart is decreased. This in turn reduces the cardiac output so that the tissues are poorly perfused. The patient's condition is usually made very much worse by the underlying pathology, e.g., peritonitis, diabetes mellitus, and the fluid lost by fever, diarrhoea, and vomiting. It is now becoming apparent that the effects produced are not due to adrenal failure caused by the endotoxins, in fact unless the adrenals are destroyed the secretion of hydrocortisone is increased.

Many conditions predispose to 'bacteriaemic shock' either by allowing organisms to enter the circulation, e.g., genito-urinary instrumentation and operations, gastrointestinal surgery, and intravenous infusions, or by reducing the body's defences, e.g., diabetes mellitus, cirrhosis, and haematological disorders.

SYMPTOMS

The patient is usually middle-aged or elderly and has

been in hospital. The onset is fairly rapid with:

i. *Rigors.*

ii. *Nausea and vomiting.*

iii. Diarrhoea.

SIGNS

i. *Tachycardia.*

ii. *Hypotension.* A fall in blood-pressure below 100 mm. Hg or more than 50 mm. Hg in a hypertensive patient is highly suspicious.

iii. *Disordered cerebration*, e.g., lethargy and confusion.

iv. Intermittent pyrexia.

v. Hyperventilation.

vi. Oliguria which develops rapidly and may progress to acute renal failure.

vii. Jaundice.

viii. Widespread purpura.

INVESTIGATIONS

i. Blood examinations.

a. Haemoglobin falls because of red blood-cell destruction.

b. White blood-count shows a polymorpholeucocytosis although a leucopenia may be present in the early stages.

c. Blood-urea rises.

d. Acid-base studies show a fall in CO_2-combining power.

e. Blood-cultures. Both aerobic and anaerobic cultures must be taken immediately the condition is suspected.

ii. *Central venous pressure.* This helps to distinguish 'bacteriaemic shock' from myocardial infarction, pulmonary embolism, and hypovolaemic shock which are the main differential diagnoses. The C.V.P. is usually normal in 'bacteriaemic shock' and either raised or lowered in the other conditions.

iii. E.C.G.

ST segment abnormalities occur because of the accompanying myocardial ischaemia.

TREATMENT

Treatment must be started immediately the diagnosis is suspected and before the blood-cultures have been read —this is the only way the mortality of this serious condition can be reduced. During treatment the blood-pressure must be carefully monitored to assess the patient's response.

i. *Antibiotics.* Antibiotic therapy must be started as soon as blood has been taken for culture. If the organism is not known and there is no indication as to its identity the following rough guide will help:

Type of organism	Primary infective condition	Antibiotic
Gram-positive	Body wall	Cephaloridine
	Bones and joints	
Gram-negative, especially *E. coli* and proteus	Genito-urinary tract Gastro-intestinal tract	Kanamycin sulphate
Clostridium	Septic abortion	Penicillin
Pseudomonas pyocyanea	Burns	Gentamicin
	Haematological disorders	
	Connective-tissue disorders	
	Steroid therapy	

Cloxacillin or methicillin can be added to any of the above antibiotics if the prescence of a hospital staphylococcus has to be considered.

ii. *Treatment of the underlying pathology.* Effectiveness in this greatly influences the mortality of the condition.

iii. *Intravenous fluids* to correct dehydration and to raise the C.V.P. to 10–15 cm. saline. Plasma-volume expanders are given when necessary.

If the blood-pressure and urinary output are not improved after this then intravenous isoprenaline should be given (2 ml. isoprenaline in 500 ml. solution given at

1 ml. per minute). The pulse-rate should be kept below 110 per minute and overdosage can be recognized by the appearance of extrasystoles on the E.C.G.

iv. Analgesics.

v. Steroids. In Gram-negative 'bacteriaemic shock' intravenous hydrocortisone (50 mg. per kg. per day at 3–6 hourly intervals for 24–36 hours) has some beneficial effect.

vi. Renal dialysis if severe renal failure develops.

F. CARDIAC ARREST

As cardiac arrest leads rapidly to respiratory failure and vice versa, attempts at resuscitation must be directed to correcting both factors. The commonest causes of cardiac arrest include myocardial anoxia following respiratory obstruction, severe haemorrhage, or massive pulmonary embolism; and toxic effects on the myocardium by drugs such as chloroform and cyclopropane. These produce a loss of cardiac function by either asystole or ventricular fibrillation. An E.C.G. recording is therefore required early in the treatment to demonstrate the state of the heart muscle.

Within seconds of being faced with a cardiac arrest the clinician must establish the diagnosis, assess the period of arrest, and decide whether or not resuscitative measures should be carried out. There is nothing to be gained by attempting resuscitation if the pupils are fixed and dilated or it is believed that the patient has been dead for more than 5 minutes. Cerebral anoxia soon develops and irreversible brain damage occurs within this period. It is also mischievous to revive patients with terminal disease unless there is an excellent reason for doing so.

Although the initial management can be performed by one person, a team of three is needed to carry out resuscitation efficiently. One member must take charge and act as leader directing and co-ordinating the various stages according to the patient's responses. He should also decide when the efforts should cease. Each member is responsible for one of the following:

i. Establishment and maintenance of an airway.

ii. External cardiac massage.

iii. Monitoring the patient and medication.

The diagnosis of cardiac arrest is confirmed by:

i. *Absent arterial pulsation*, which is checked by feeling for a femoral pulse at the groin. The carotid pulse should not be used as pressure on it may jeopardize an already critical blood-supply to the brain.

ii. *Absent or gasping respirations.*

iii. *Dilating or dilated pupils.* Dilatation of the pupils begins about 45 seconds after the heart stops and is complete after 2 minutes.

MANAGEMENT

i. Establishment and maintenance of an airway. This takes precedence over all other procedures which are wasted if oxygen cannot reach the lungs.

a. Clear airway. Check that the airway is not blocked by mucus, blood, vomit, or the tongue. Extend the neck and hold up the chin.

b. Endotracheal intubation. This is the most efficient method of ensuring a completely satisfactory ventilatory system but requires some skill to carry out. While waiting for endotracheal intubation to be performed mouth-to-mouth respiration with an airway of the Brook type is sufficient.

c. Mechanical ventilation. An oxygen mask placed over the face of the patient is useless when treating this condition. Positive-pressure ventilation by either mouth-to-mouth breathing, a bag and mask, or a machine must be used and the lungs inflated at a rate of between ten and twenty times each minute.

d. Oxygen. The flow rate for adults is 8–10 litres per

minute and for children 6–8 litres per minute.

ii. External cardiac massage. External cardiac massage has superseded internal (open) cardiac massage which is now only used if the chest is already open or when severe thoracic trauma is present.

a. Firm surface. The patient should be lying on a firm surface, e.g., a board under the mattress of the bed or on the floor.

b. Pressure on the sternum. The operator places his hands one on top of the other over the lower sternum and sharply exerts sufficient pressure to push the sternum inwards for 4–5 cm. (2·5 cm. for a child). The pressure is released and the movement repeated approximately sixty times a minute. Vigorous pressure is rarely required unless the rib cage is unyielding as in severe emphysema.

The heel of the lower hand must remain on the sternum during each stroke. If it strays on to the rib cage the heart will not receive sufficient compression and there is also a risk of fracturing the ribs which may then pierce the underlying structures.

iii. Monitoring the patient and medication.

Palpation of the femoral pulsation will suffice until an E.C.G. can be set up.

a. E.C.G. This must be set up as soon as possible to decide whether asystole or ventricular fibrillation is present and then to check the response of the patient to treatment.

b. Intravenous infusion. Time must not be wasted trying to set up a drip in the routine manner. If an intravenous infusion is not already in position, a cannula should be passed percutaneously into the subclavian vein (*see* p. 101) or, if this is impracticable, a cut-down performed using the long saphenous vein at the ankle.

c. Drugs. These are administered by either an intravenous infusion or directly into the heart. When an injection is made into the heart it must be into the ventricle cavity and not into the ventricle wall where it may produce an irritable focus and cause fibrillation. Drugs are used to correct the following problems:

1. Tissue acidosis: sodium bicarbonate is given to treat the tissue acidosis produced by hypoxia. The dose is 40–50 mmol. by intravenous infusion every 15 minutes.

2. Asystole: adrenaline—10 ml. of a 1 : 10,000 solution—injected directly into the heart should produce ventricular fibrillation which is then treated as such.

3. Ventricular fibrillation: either calcium chloride, 10 ml. of a 5–10 per cent solution, or lignocaine, 25–75 mg., is effective in suppressing the irritability of the heart. Lignocaine is also given as a constant intravenous infusion (1–4 mg. per minute) after successful defibrillation.

4. Hypotension: Metaraminol (Aramine) 50 mg. in 500 ml. normal saline. The rate of infusion is regulated to maintain the blood-pressure at an acceptable level once a normal rhythm has resumed.

d. *Defibrillation* (by trained personnel only). When ventricular fibrillation occurs a defibrillating current is required to revert it to sinus rhythm.

e. *Treatment of the primary cause of the cardiac arrest*, e.g., correct haemorrhage, electrolyte disturbance, drug toxicity, etc.

After successful resuscitation the incidence of recurrent cardiac arrest is high and the patient should be carefully monitored for at least 24 hours. Management during this period includes:

1. Continuous E.C.G. recording.

2. Support of respiration if necessary.

3. Give 200 ml. of 20 per cent mannitol. It is often useful to catheterize the bladder to check the urinary output.

4. X-ray of the chest to look for fractured ribs or a pneumothorax that may have been produced by the cardiac massage.

Chapter 8

Practical procedures

An intravenous infusion can be set up by percutaneous venepuncture or a formal cut-down. The majority of these procedures are carried out by percutaneous venepuncture and a cut-down reserved for occasions when venepuncture is impracticable, for cases of cardiac arrest, and when parenteral feeding is required for a long period. Both procedures are relatively simple to perform but practice is required to obtain real proficiency.

When selecting a site for giving an intravenous infusion the upper limb should be the first choice and the lower limb avoided because of the increased risks of thrombophlebitis and deep-vein thrombosis. However, there are two exceptions to this generalization. In cardiac arrest a cut-down at the ankle is more convenient as it can be carried out quickly without interfering with those personnel maintaining cardiac and respiratory function. Another exception is long-term parenteral feeding when tributaries of the long saphenous vein may be cannulated in the groin.

The selection of the vein is important. A fairly straight vein away from any joint is advised as the needle will have to be advanced along the lumen of the vein for a distance of 1–2 cm., and movement of a nearby joint could cause the vein to tear with leakage of fluid. When drugs, irritant solutions such as dextrose, and fluids for parenteral nutrition are to be infused only large veins should be used as phlebitis and leakage of fluid occur very quickly with small veins.

The site most frequently used for a cut-down is the cephalic vein where it lies quite superficially in the arm just lateral to the body of the biceps brachialis. It rarely becomes thrombosed even when repeated intravenous infusions have been previously placed in the forearm. The cephalic vein can also be found in the deltopectoral groove, but in this position it frequently lies hidden between the borders of the two muscles. In cases of cardiac arrest the long saphenous vein can be found 1 cm. above and anterior to the medial malleolus and cannulated with a large-bore catheter.

With both methods of setting up an intravenous infusion an aseptic technique is mandatory if complications resulting from the presence of the cannula are to be kept to a minimum. The commonest complications include:

i. Phlebitis. This is usually a chemical inflammation caused by the presence of the cannula in the vein. It produces local pain, swelling, and erythema but rarely causes thrombosis with embolism. When phlebitis occurs the cannula must be removed immediately and warm packs applied to the part. The practice of leaving the drip in situ and treating the lesion with solutions such as glycerin and ichthyol is to be abhorred by any sensible clinician.

ii. Septicaemia. It has been estimated that nearly a half of all hospital-acquired septicaemias originate from the site of an intravenous infusion. Most of the cases follow the prolonged use of a plastic cannula, e.g., for monitoring the central venous pressure, or a cut-down which has been performed hastily with a lack of aseptic technique. The causative organisms either pass along the outside of the cannula by capillary attraction or are introduced into the infusion fluid when extra electrolytes, etc., are added.

When local inflammation, unexplained sepsis, or a swinging temperature suggests a septicaemia the catheter must be removed at once and cultures taken from the tip of the cannula and blood. Antibiotics are given and changed only if the bacterial cultures show the presence of resistant organisms. Fungal infections have also been reported with intravenous catheters and must be borne in mind.

iii. Embolization of catheter material. When using percutaneous needle-catheter units precautions must be taken to ensure that the needle cannot inadvertently divide the cannula, e.g., by sliding a protective plastic sleeve over the point of the needle where the cannula emerges.

Explicit instructions must be given regarding the infusion rate, the total volume to be given, and the amounts of drugs and electrolytes, etc., that are to be added to the fluid.

RAPID INFUSIONS

In certain emergencies such as severe acute blood-loss the intravenous fluid must be given very quickly and either several drips can be set up simultaneously or a method used to pump the fluid into the vein using a positive pressure. A positive pressure in the fluid bottle can be produced by attaching a Higginson's syringe to its outflow tube, but as this method has been responsible for many fatal cases of air embolism it should only be used as a last resort. Instead one of the more acceptable and less risky methods should be used and even then the clinician must be present all the time it is in use and only the initial three-quarters of the fluid in each bottle should be given under pressure.

i. If the fluid to be given is in a collapsible plastic container then squeezing the container will increase the flow of fluid through the infusion set.

ii. The drip chamber of many plastic infusion sets contains a ball which allows fluid to be given quickly by manually squeezing the drip chamber (*Fig. 2*). Compressing the drip chamber forces fluid into the vein under pressure and when the chamber is empty the ball

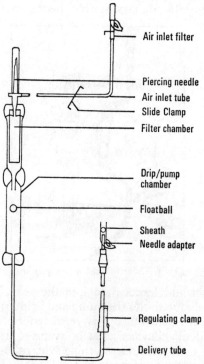

Fig. 2.—Drip chamber. (*By courtesy of Baxter Division, Travenol Laboratories Ltd., Thetford, Norfolk.*) To use the pump chamber for a pressure transfusion (this should only be carried out under the constant supervision of a doctor, and discontinued when the bottle is empty): (i) Close regulating clamp and squeeze lower pump chamber to fill completely so that the floatball occludes the inlet. (ii) Open the regulating clamp and alternately squeeze and release the pump chamber allowing it to fill completely between each action.

occludes the exit. As the chamber returns to its normal shape fluid is drawn in to fill it again. To prevent the fluid returning to the reservoir during this procedure the ball occludes the inlet during the compression.

iii. The Martin's pump (*Fig.* 3) consists of rollers which compress the collapsible plastic tubing of the

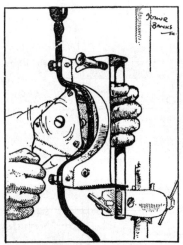

Fig. 3.—Martin's roller pump in use.

infusion set and forces fluid into the vein. The tubing can be easily fitted into the pump and held firmly in place by clips. The rate of flow is regulated by turning the handle and the clinician must be aware of the risk of air embolism if he continues turning when the reservoir is empty. The pump must not be used if the plastic tubing has been punctured by giving intravenous injections into it as air can be sucked in to produce air embolism.

CENTRAL VENOUS PRESSURE (C.V.P.) MEASUREMENT

Since its clinical introduction in 1952 the measurement of C.V.P. has gained increasing popularity as a method of obtaining continuous information about cardiac function. It is a measurement of the pressure in the region of the right atrium and adjacent portions of both venae cavae, thereby demonstrating how the heart is dealing with returning venous blood. It does not measure the blood-volume but is an extremely useful guide to fluid replacement in severely ill and hypovolaemic patients.

Care must be taken when interpreting the results as they are very susceptible to errors. There is a wide range of normal values which is reported as varying between 0 and 12 cm. water, but for patients with chronic pulmonary disease the accepted 'normal value' may be 16 cm. water or more. However, when used sensibly repeated measurements of the C.V.P. give an indication as to the response of the heart to changes in blood-volume, etc. For example, a fall in C.V.P. could indicate:

i. Loss of blood-volume, e.g., haemorrhage or dehydration.

ii. Increased cardiac efficiency, e.g., digitalis therapy.

iii. Impaired venous return to the chest, e.g., ascites or acute gastric dilatation.

Whereas a rise in C.V.P. could indicate:

i. Overloading of the circulation.

ii. Heart failure.

iii. Raised intrathoracic pressure, e.g., cardiac tamponade, pleural effusion, haemo- or pneumothorax.

Techniques for setting up a C.V.P. Line

Several sites and methods have been recommended and each has its advocates.

i. *Subclavian vein* (infraclavicular approach). In order to ensure long-term catheter sterility and the minimum of complications a full aseptic technique must be used and the patient either completely unconscious or fully co-operative.

a. Elevate the foot of the bed, so that the patient is in the Trendelenburg position. This distends the sub-clavian vein and also reduces the risk of complications from air embolism.

b. The skin is cleaned and local anaesthetic injected if required.

c. A 14-gauge Intracath needle is attached to a 10-ml. syringe.

d. The needle is introduced through the skin 1 cm. below and just medial to the mid-point of the right clavicle. Using the right side avoids damage to the thoracic duct. From this point gentle suction must be maintained by the syringe to prevent air being sucked into the vein as the pressure in the vein is low and this is accentuated by hypovolaemic states. If the suction is too vigorous the vein wall may collapse.

e. The needle is pushed parallel to the chest wall and directed towards the space between the sternal and clavicular heads of the sternomastoid muscle. The return of venous blood indicates successful puncture of the vein.

f. If the patient is conscious he should now inspire deeply and hold his breath. This manœuvre increases the venous pressure and reduces the risk of air embolism during the next stage.

g. The syringe is removed and a flexible radio-opaque intravenous catheter is quickly threaded through the needle for about 5 cm. The needle is withdrawn from the skin and the catheter aspirated to check back-flow of blood. The catheter is then secured and attached to the manometer. An antibiotic cream is placed around the puncture site.

ii. *Internal jugular vein.* The internal jugular vein is constant in position, lying attached to the deep surface of the sternomastoid just lateral to the mid-point of the muscle. The carotid artery lies medial and deep to the vein. Percutaneous puncture of the right internal jugular vein is easy to perform on a patient under a general anaesthetic and the procedure produces very few complications.

a. Using positive-pressure ventilation the patient is tilted in a head-down position and the head turned to the left. The vein distends to a diameter of approximately 2·5 cm. and is usually palpable. It can be distinguished easily from the carotid artery.

b. The skin is cleaned, and full aseptic technique used.

c. A 14-gauge Intracath needle is attached to a 10-ml. syringe.

d. Gentle suction is maintained on the syringe as the needle is introduced at an angle of about 40° to the skin at a point where the vein is easily palpable. It is then advanced posteriorly, laterally, and caudally through the deep fascia into the vein. As the needle passes through the fascia and vein wall there is a definite click and a reflux of venous blood.

e. The syringe is removed and a flexible radio-opaque intravenous catheter is quickly threaded through the needle for about 5 cm. A large catheter is used for adults and most children and a medium catheter for newborn infants and small children.

f. The needle is withdrawn and a swab applied firmly to the puncture site. An antibiotic cream is placed around the puncture site.

The first method is easy and quick to carry out on the fully conscious co-operative patient and the second method is very useful for the patient under a general anaesthetic. Other methods include the percutaneous puncture of the external jugular vein or the cephalic vein in the arm or antecubital fossa.

Complications of Cannulation for measuring C.V.P.

i. Thrombophlebitis. This occurs in between 20 and 40 per cent of all cases after 48 hours. The lowest incidence is found when the internal jugular vein is used and by far the highest incidence occurs with percutaneous puncture of the cephalic vein.

ii. Septicaemia. This occurs in 2–2·5 per cent of all patients after 48 hours.

iii. Pneumothorax or haemothorax. This occurs in 0·2–2·0 per cent of all cases and the majority follow cannulation of the subclavian vein. Although it is usually an immediate complication it occasionally occurs as a late development. The patient complains of chest pain and dyspnoea and on examination the breath-sounds are found to be unequal. Once a chest X-ray has confirmed the diagnosis, closed chest drainage is instituted. It is therefore important to examine the chest of every unconscious patient who has had this procedure carried out.

This complication occurs most often in obese and uncooperative patients and in these cases it is often easier to cut down on the cephalic vein in the deltopectoral groove or use a very long Intracath introduced at the elbow (antecubital fossa).

iv. Air embolism. It is almost inevitable that small quantities of air will enter the veins during this procedure, but they should not reach a harmful amount if the technique is carried out correctly.

v. Cardiac tamponade. This will occur if the cannula penetrates the heart wall and can be avoided by accurately locating the tip of the cannula in the superior vena cava and not forcing the passage of the cannula.

Other complications that may occur include catheter embolus when the cannula breaks off, arteriovenous fistulae, brachial plexus palsy, and massive cutaneous emphysema which may require a tracheostomy.

Measurement of C.V.P.

The ruler must be zeroed at the level of the right atrium and different methods are used for finding this point.

i. Three to four cm. below the sternal angle when the patient is upright. The sternal angle is the point where the manubrium sterni joins the body of the sternum.

ii. Ten cm. above the table or bed when the patient is lying flat.

iii. At either the anterior axillary line or the mid-axillary line when the patient is lying flat.

The reference point decided upon for any particular patient must be noted and used for further measurements even though the position of the patient may be changed. It is also important that positive-pressure breathing should be disconnected when measuring C.V.P.

URETHRAL CATHETERIZATION

The indication for the majority of catheterizations carried out as emergency procedures is acute retention of urine. However, emergency catheterization can also be required for irrigation of the bladder with antibacterial agents, the removal of blood-clots, or for applying pressure to the prostate gland or prostatic bed when they are bleeding, e.g., to obtain haemostasis after a prostatectomy.

The type of catheter used tends to be a matter of personal choice, but the decision is usually influenced by the age and sex of the patient and the reason for the procedure. Catheters are graded according to size and the Charrière (French) scale is the one most commonly used. In this scale the sizes represent the circumference or three times the diameter of the catheter in millimetres. For conversion of this scale to one of the three others that may be used the following formula is employed:

Charrière scale × 2 = (English scale × 3) + 6 = American scale × 3 = Béniqué scale, e.g., catheter 5 mm. diameter = 15 C (Fg) = 8 E = 10 A = 30 B.

Large catheters (16–10 Fg) are easy to introduce and cause very little trauma to the adult urethra. Also they are firm enough not to coil up in the urethra when they meet resistance at the external sphincter. Small catheters (approximately 10 Fg) are necessary for children, and infants require even smaller catheters (6 Fg). The narrowest part of the normal urethra is the external urinary meatus and catheters that can pass this point should be able to pass along the whole length of a normal urethra.

TECHNIQUE

The procedure should be explained to the patient so that he understands what it involves and what to expect. The pubic area must be shaved and the subsequent steps carried out with a strict aseptic technique. The catheter is only handled with sterile forceps supplied for this specific purpose.

i. The patient is placed on his back with his hips abducted and slightly flexed.

ii. The area is cleaned and the foreskin retracted to enable its undersurface to be cleaned. Preparations containing alcohol should not be used for cleaning as they have an irritant effect on the urethral mucosa. Sterile towels are then arranged so that only the penis is exposed. The penis is wrapped in a sterile gauze swab.

iii. Five ml. of an antiseptic cream, e.g., 5 per cent Hibitane in glycerin, is introduced into the urethra with a syringe. When a local anaesthetic agent, e.g., 2 per cent lignocaine cream, is used it must be placed in the urethra before the antiseptic cream.

iv. The distal 10 cm. of the catheter is lubricated with sterile liquid paraffin.

v. The penis held vertically so that the urethra is converted from an S shape to a C shape.

vi. The catheter is advanced slowly but firmly along the urethra until the slight resistance of the external sphincter is felt. At this point the patient takes a few deep breaths and the catheter should slip easily into the bladder. This will be confirmed by the passage of urine along the catheter.

Catheterization is easier in women than men as the female urethra is only 3–4 cm. in length. The woman is placed in the lithotomy position and the labia held apart so that the urethral opening is clearly seen.

vii. The catheter is connected to a closed drainage system and either securely strapped to the patient or held in place by a self-retaining balloon.

If the catheter fails to enter the bladder a smaller catheter can be tried. If this attempt is also unsuccessful then the procedure should be abandoned and someone with more experience called. Persistence or forceful pushing with the catheter leads to trauma and bleeding which make further attempts more difficult and greatly increases the problems encountered during management of the patient.

When the bladder has been chronically distended the decompression should be carried out slowly allowing only 100 ml. of urine to escape from the bladder every hour. Too rapid a decompression produces bleeding from the submucosal blood-vessels as the oedematous mucosa is unable to contract as efficiently as the muscle wall and is sheared off the submucosa. The bleeding can be very severe and clot retention often occurs.

COMPLICATIONS

i. Infection. Bacteria enter the bladder either by passing along the lumen of the catheter or through urethral secretions which, if unable to escape from the urethra, form a crust which provides a culture medium for bacteria. In order to reduce the incidence of infection narrow-bore catheters made of a non-irritant substance, e.g., polyvinyl chloride, are used and attached to a closed-circuit drainage with as few connexions as possible. Any strapping used to fix the catheter should allow free escape of urethral secretions from the external urinary meatus. Disconnexion of the circuit at any time or the need for recatheterization should be rigorously avoided.

ii. Urethral stricture. This is a later complication and can follow a traumatic catheterization or occur when a large catheter has been left in place for too long a period.

Chapter 9

Intravenous fluids

Intravenous fluids are used during the management of surgical emergencies.

i. To replace blood-volume.

ii. For correcting some anaemias.

iii. To give fluid or nutrient materials when oral or tube feeding is impracticable.

iv. To promote an osmotic diuresis.

A loss of blood-volume occurs when one or more of the components of blood is lost from the body during a relatively short period of time. After the immediate generalized vasoconstriction the body attempts to replace the loss by moving fluid from the tissues into the circulation. If these mechanisms are insufficient to maintain renal perfusion the production of aldosterone and anti-diuretic hormone is increased and further loss of fluid through the kidneys as urine is prevented. The components of the blood-volume that may be lost either together or individually are:

i. *Extracellular fluid.* Large quantities of extracellular fluid can be lost from the gastro-intestinal tract as vomit and diarrhoea or, less obviously, into the lumen of obstructed bowel. This fluid contains approximately the same concentrations of sodium and chloride as blood (*Table* 5), and when there is a severe depletion of water and sodium chloride a potassium deficiency follows. Fluid lost by these methods must therefore be replaced with isotonic (0.9 per cent) saline in volumes equal to the amount lost. If large quantities of fluid are required in a short period of time a more accurate plasma ratio of 140 Na : 100 Cl can be maintained by adding 1 litre of sodium lactate or sodium bicarbonate to every 2 litres of isotonic saline given.

Table 5. MEAN ELECTROLYTE CONTENT OF GASTRO-INTESTINAL SECRETIONS AND SERUM

	CONCENTRATION (mmol/l.)		
	Na$^+$	K$^+$	Cl$^-$
Gastric	60	9·5	100
Biliary	145	5·5	100
Pancreatic	140	5·0	75
Small intestinal	120	5·0	100
Serum	135–140	3·5–5·0	98–106

Extracellular fluid is also lost during the postoperative period by patients who are unable to take fluids orally. This loss occurs relatively slowly and the routine use of intravenous therapy following abdominal surgery, etc., has made any ill effects from this loss a rarity. After surgery or trauma the body retains sodium and excretes potassium in the urine for a period of time that varies with the degree of tissue damage. This response lasts for at least 24 hours and during this time fluid balance can be maintained by an infusion of 5 per cent dextrose, adding 1 litre of isotonic saline every 24 hours after the first day.

The daily fluid requirements of individual patients during the postoperative period vary but a reasonable assessment can be made by totalling up the measurable fluid loss from the body as urine and gastric aspiration, etc., and adding to it 800 ml. for 'insensible loss'. For an otherwise healthy, fit adult 2 litres during the first 24 hours and 3 litres during each subsequent 24 hours are usually sufficient.

ii. *Plasma.* Large quantities of plasma are lost from the body surface of patients with burns and into the peritoneal cavity of patients with peritonitis or acute pancreatitis.

iii. *Blood.* Acute blood-loss may be obvious, e.g., haematemesis and melaena, or hidden, e.g., ruptured spleen and ischaemic bowel.

If loss of blood-volume is allowed to continue unchecked peripheral circulatory failure and death eventually occur. In such cases replacement of blood-volume is imperative and whenever possible the particular component lost should be given. Factors which help in deciding the amount and type of fluid lost include:

HISTORY

An accurate history of the symptoms and their duration must be obtained.

SIGNS

A minimum of 3 litres of fluid must be lost to produce obvious clinical signs of dehydration in an adult.

i. *Diminished skin elasticity.* Allowances must be made for similar changes in skin elasticity found with advancing age and recent weight-loss.

ii. *Reduced urinary output.*

iii. Pallor and empty veins.

iv. Dry mouth (allow for mouth breathing) and dry conjunctivae.

v. Coldness of the extremities.

vi. Increasing pulse-rate.

vii. Hypotension.

INVESTIGATIONS

i. Haemoglobin and P.C.V.

ii. Blood-urea and electrolytes.

A rough guide to changes of (i) and (ii):

Type of fluid lost	Hb	Investigation P.C.V.	Urea
Extracellular fluid	Progressive rise	Progressive rise	Increases
Plasma	Increases	Increases	Increases
Blood	Progressive fall	Progressive fall	Increases

iii. Central venous pressure.
iv. Urinary measurements.

With the loss of blood-volume urinary output is reduced, its specific gravity increased, and there is a decreased excretion of sodium.

These investigations are repeated regularly during treatment and guide further fluid replacement. Measurement of the central venous pressure is essential when fluid replacement is to be carried out rapidly in elderly patients or patients whose cardiac state is doubtful. In an otherwise normal patient a rapid infusion of 500 ml. every 15 minutes can be tolerated without harmful effect.

When an infusion remains in place for more than 24 hours the serum electrolytes should be measured daily and alterations in management carried out as indicated by the results. In some severely ill patients a low serum sodium concentration occurs and persists in spite of the administration of large amounts of sodium. This very serious condition probably results from failure of the sodium pump mechanism of the cells and is described as the 'sick-cell syndrome'.

When fluid balance has been restored the rate of urine flow should return to approximately 50–60 ml. per hour and the various parameters being measured return to normal limits.

INTRAVENOUS FLUID THERAPY IN PAEDIATRICS

The fluid requirements of premature infants and neonates, and the administration of blood or intravenous calories to children are specialist problems and will not be discussed here. However, the administration of water and electrolyte requirements to older infants and children is a more common problem and worth mentioning as inadequate fluid replacement often occurs in this group. In fact it has been shown to be a causative factor in over a third of the children who still die following acute appendicitis. In general the causes of fluid loss and dehydration are similar to those found in the adult but certain important differences do exist:

i. Extracellular fluid lost from the intestine by vomiting, etc., contains a disproportionately large amount of potassium which has to be replaced when replacing the fluid loss.

ii. The younger the child the less marked are the normal responses to trauma and the kidneys' ability to retain sodium.

iii. When a child has had the usual restriction of fluid prior to operation the fluid deficit per kg. is much larger (up to three times as great) relative to the adult patient.

DIAGNOSIS OF THE DEGREE OF DEHYDRATION IN CHILDREN

a. History.
b. Signs.

	General state	Mouth and tongue	Skin	Anterior fontanelle (*if open*)
Mild	Irritable	Dry	Flushed warm and dry	Soft
Moderate	Restless and anxious	Very dry	Reduced elasticity	Depressed
Severe	Apathetic and unresponsive	Extreme dryness	Marked loss of skin elasticity	Markedly depressed

Progressive oliguria, pyrexia, and a sunken appearance of the eyes are also noticed and are related to the degree of dehydration.

INVESTIGATIONS

a. Haemoglobin and P.C.V. These are useful but are not as reliable as in adults because of the wide range of normal values accepted in infants and young children.

b. Serum electrolytes and urea.

c. Body-weight.

d. Urinary output.

These investigations, together with clinical examination, must be repeated regularly during treatment to assess the response.

INTRAVENOUS REQUIREMENTS

Calculations regarding fluid and electrolyte requirements for children either take into consideration surface area or body-weight. The surface area is particularly important in children as it is greater in relation to body-weight than for an adult, and a greater proportion of fluid is therefore lost by 'insensible loss'. This loss depends very greatly on the temperature of the child and its environment. Unfortunately the estimation of surface area can be difficult and to add to the problem the clinician has a choice of more than thirty-seven formulae for its calculation. The régime of intravenous therapy selected will depend on whether it is for the maintenance of fluid balance or as a replacement therapy in the dehydrated child.

Maintenance

A simple method for calculating maintenance requirements according to body weight is described here. It is both easy to remember and clinically acceptable (*Table*.6).

Replacement

The commonest causes of dehydration are vomiting and diarrhoea and the replacement therapy depends upon the degree of dehydration that has occurred. If severe the low plasma volume must be first corrected by giving plasma and then isotonic (0·9 per cent) saline until the

Table 6. METHOD OF ESTIMATING FLUID MAINTENANCE
FOR A CHILD

BODY-WEIGHT	FLUID REQUIRED	Na+ or Cl−	K+
0–10 kg.	100 ml. per kg. per 24 hr.	3 mmol. per kg. per 24 hr.	2 mmol. per kg. per 24 hr.
11–20 kg.	1000 ml.+50 ml. per kg. over 10 kg. per 24 hr.	30+1·5 mmol. per kg. over 10 kg. per 24 hr.	20+1 mmol. per kg. over 10 kg. per 24 hr.
20 kg.<	1500 ml.+20 ml. per kg. over 20 kg. per 24 hr.	45+0·6 mmol. per kg. over 20 kg. per 24 hr.	30+0·4 mmol. per kg. over 20 kg. per 24 hr.

urinary output is reasonable. A solution with a high potassium content, e.g., Darrow's solution, is then given until the child regains normal clinical and biochemical hydration when maintenance therapy, such as the above régime, can be instituted. The importance of giving adequate potassium must be stressed as the deficiency is usually greater than suspected and its measurement as a guide to replacement is unreliable.

BLOOD
A transfusion of blood may be required during the management of surgical emergencies for:

i. Replacement of acute blood-loss or to restore a normal level after chronic blood-loss.

ii. Severe infections. As blood formation is depressed blood must be given to help the patient deal effectively with the infection.

iii. Bleeding diatheses when factors missing from the patient's blood can be replaced by transfusions of fresh blood.

REACTIONS TO BLOOD TRANSFUSIONS

Blood should not be given to a patient unless there is a clear indication as reactions to blood transfusion are a common problem and disastrous results can occur if they are not recognized and treated immediately. In all cases the patient's identity must be double checked against the data on the blood container, and signs of reaction must be carefully watched for during the first 100 ml. infusion.

i. *Simple pyrexial reactions.* A mild pyrexia during a transfusion is common but it poses a problem for the clinician who must decide whether or not to stop the transfusion. Patients vary in their tendency to develop this reaction, but it often occurs in patients who have had a previous transfusion. As long as the temperature remains below 38·3 C. (101° F.) and there are no other adverse signs and symptoms the transfusion can be cautiously continued. Aspirin may be given to settle the pyrexia but no other treatment is advised as it may mask the onset of more serious reactions.

ii. *Allergic transfusion reactions.* These reactions to transfused foreign protein are rare (less than 1 per cent transfusions), but when they occur there is often a past history of allergic conditions, e.g., asthma, hay fever, or allergic reaction to a transfusion. Characteristically the symptoms present towards the end of the transfusion or after its completion and all grades of severity can occur.

If minimal the patient complains of itching and urticaria. This is not serious and apart from slowing down the rate of transfusion and reviewing the patient at regular intervals no specific treatment is required. The reaction usually subsides spontaneously after 2–6 hours. When severe, the reaction starts with rigors or fever and may proceed to facial or laryngeal oedema with bronchial spasm. The transfusion must be stopped immediately and antihistamine drugs, e.g., promethazine hydrochloride (Phenergan) or chlorpheniramine maleate (Piriton), given intramuscularly or by slow intravenous injection.

iii. *Bacterial contamination of blood*. There is always a risk that blood may become contaminated during withdrawal from the donor but the organisms are usually destroyed by defence mechanisms in the fresh blood. Any bacteria that survive may be prevented from multiplying by storing the blood at 4° C. However, certain organisms, e.g., *Escherichia coli* and *Pseudomonas*, can survive and either grow at this temperature or multiply rapidly once the blood is removed from refrigeration. To minimize this risk blood should not be left at room temperature for more than 30 minutes on any one occasion before use and preparations of concentrated red cells must be used as soon as possible and certainly not more than 12 hours after preparation.

Blood contaminated with *E. coli* and *Pseudomonas*, etc., is usually easily recognized by the pathologist carrying out the cross-match, but any blood with an unusual appearance should be discarded by the clinician. Normal blood has a clear line of demarcation between the settled red cells and plasma and if the plasma is reddish-purple and not straw-coloured then haemolysins are present.

If infected blood is given to a patient either bacteriaemic shock or a miliary type of infection occurs. After starting the transfusion the patient becomes ill very quickly with flushing, headache, vomiting, diarrhoea, hypotension, hyperpyrexia, or a massive bleeding diathesis. The transfusion must be stopped immediately and the blood cultured. Further treatment is as for bacteriaemic shock, but the prognosis is poor.

iv. *Reaction to an incompatible transfusion.* The effects produced by an incompatible transfusion vary considerably but, by and large, depend on the amount of blood given and the state of the body's normal responses. For example, the earlier a reaction is noted during a transfusion the more serious it tends to be and the greater are the morbidity and mortality. Some of the more moderate reactions may be undiagnosed if the clinician is not constantly aware of their presentation. Sometimes the donor's red cells are not destroyed in the blood-stream but in the reticulo-endothelial system and very few symptoms and signs are observed. Only a small amount of free haemoglobin is liberated and the reaction may only be suspected when a rise in serum bilirubin occurs or the expected rise in haemoglobin after transfusion does not occur.

When incompatible blood is given during an operation the only signs of a haemolytic reaction may be unexplained hypotension or sudden, spontaneous, diffuse bleeding from the tissues. The bleeding is produced by a form of defibrination syndrome and, although the specific treatment depends on identifying the specific defect, satisfactory results can be obtained by a transfusion of 300–500 ml. fresh frozen plasma and 4 g. of fibrinogen intravenously which is repeated if necessary. When clot lysis is observed on testing, ε-amino-caproic acid should be given intravenously in 2–4-g. doses.

More obvious haemolytic transfusion reactions present with the well-known symptoms and signs of pyrexia, lumbar or chest pain, faintness, nausea, headache, flushing of the face, rigors, blood-stained urine, or hypotension. The most serious cases are heralded by rigors, fever, and acute circulatory collapse. Free haemoglobin is present in the urine and in these cases prompt treatment is required to save the patient's life and prevent permanent renal damage.

INVESTIGATIONS

i. Check the details of the patient with the labels on the blood bottle.

ii. Haemoglobin.

iii. All the urine passed by the patient must be examined. A low output or a persistent S.G. below 1·010 indicates renal damage.

iv. Urine haemoglobin.

v. Samples of the donor blood must be rechecked against a pretransfusion sample from the recipient.

vi. Direct antiglobulin (Coombs) test on the recipient red cells.

vii. The patient's serum must also be checked for atypical or incomplete antibody. After prolonged treatment with certain drugs, e.g. methyldopa (Aldomet), a specific auto-antibody may be found so details of drug history must be given to the pathologist.

viii. Gram stain and culture of the remaining blood in the blood bottle.

TREATMENT

i. Stop the transfusion.

ii. Treat any circulatory failure.

iii. When anuria occurs treat the renal failure.

iv. Any bleeding diathesis is treated as described.

v. *Citrate and potassium poisoning.* Citrate is rapidly metabolized by the liver and toxic effects due to its excess only occur during exchange transfusions in infants whose liver is not fully functional or following massive transfusions to adults with a degree of liver failure. It causes tremors of the skeletal muscles and a marked prolongation of the S–T segment on the E.C.G. Treatment in the adult is by a slow intravenous injection of 10 ml. of 10 per cent calcium gluconate (and proportionately less to an infant). The dose is repeated after every second bottle of blood in long continuous transfusions.

When blood is stored, potassium is lost from the red cells into the plasma. Fresh plasma contains 4–5 mmol. potassium per litre but this rises to about 15 mmol. per litre after storage for 10 days and reaches 20 mmol. per litre after 20 days. It follows that a massive transfusion of stored blood will produce a rise in the recipient's circulating potassium level. If this level reaches 8 mmol. per litre changes in the E.C.G. will be observed, e.g., Q–T segment prolongation, bradycardia, and irregularities of the rhythm; and when it reaches 10 mmol. per litre ventricular fibrillation with cardiac arrest occurs.

vi. *Overloading of the circulation.* It is relatively easy to overtransfuse patients particularly when chronic anaemia or cardiac failure are present and judgement is required in determining the amount and rate of replacement of blood-volume. When the excess fluid is able to escape from the circulation, e.g., saline, pulmonary oedema results but infused blood remains producing overdistension of the circulation. The patient may complain of a persistent cough, frothy and sometimes blood-stained sputum, or dyspnoea. The veins of the neck become distended and râles are heard in the chest.

TREATMENT

i. Stop the transfusion.

ii. Morphine 15 mg. and atropine 1 mg. subcutaneously.

iii. Venesection or the application of tourniquets to the limbs.

iv. Oxygen.

v. Diuretics.

The transfusion of massive volumes of unwarmed blood causes a significant loss of heat from the tissues thereby increasing the risk of acidosis and failure of the liver to metabolize citrate. This blood should be warmed before infusion but it is unnecessary and even unwise to warm blood bottles routinely before the transfusion.

Warming can easily result in overheating which damages the red cells and if there is delay before the blood is given bacterial growth may occur.

When blood needs to be warmed to body temperature special methods should be used. These include passage through a disposable plastic coil immersed in a controlled water-bath or a radio-frequency induction bottle heater.

Warmed unused blood must be discarded and not returned to the blood bank.

PLASMA

Plasma is valuable for the emergency replacement of blood-volume as it can be given without delay. Dried plasma can be kept at room temperature for an unlimited period and is reconstituted by shaking and mixing with sterile pyrogen-free distilled water. It is given by an intravenous infusion which can be as rapid as 3 bottles (1·7 litres) in 30 minutes but except in special circumstances only 2 bottles (1·1 litres) should be given to a patient at any one time. Unfortunately plasma carries a small risk of causing virus hepatitis.

DEXTRAN

Dextran was developed as a plasma substitute and has proved a very effective and safe means of replacing blood-volume without carrying the risk of transmitting hepatitis. Four solutions of different molecular weight are manufactured by the action of certain bacteria on sucrose phosphate. The average molecular weight of the solution is indicated in its name, e.g., dextran 70 has an approximate molecular weight of 70,000. The length of time a dextran remains in the circulation is related to its molecular weight, but the use of the large molecular weight dextrans, e.g., 110 and 150, is limited as they produce red-cell aggregation and interfere with the cross-matching of blood. Any blood required for cross-matching must be taken before giving any dextran solution. Dextran may be dangerous in patients with severe congestive heart failure, renal failure, or coagulation defects.

Dextran 70 (Dextraven 70, Macrodex) will give a reliable blood-volume over many hours and also has marked antithrombotic properties. In hypovolaemic shock a litre of dextran 70 may be given and although the dextran has no oxygen-carrying power some degree of haemodilution at a haematocrit of 30 per cent actually increases the capacity of blood to transport oxygen. If further replacement of blood-volume is required then blood should be given. Dextran also reduces the thrombo-embolic complications of hypovolaemic shock.

Dextran 70 has also been used to prevent deep-vein thrombosis in patients of the high-risk groups who are undergoing surgery. Five hundred ml. are given during the operation and on the first postoperative day. It is then given every other day for as long as the patient is considered to be at risk.

Dextran 40 (Lomodex, Rheomacrodex) is primarily used for improving blood-flow and preventing rouleaux formation (sludging) of red blood-cells rather than expanding blood-volume as the solution leaves the body through the kidneys within a few hours.

PARENTERAL NUTRITION

Following trauma and stress the body produces non-specific responses which cause an increased utilization of calories by the tissues. As many surgical patients also have the effects of starvation superimposed upon this catabolic response the small stores of glycogen in the liver are soon exhausted and tissue protein has to be broken down to supply carbohydrate residues for metabolism and amino-acids for repair of damaged tissues. This results in an increased loss of nitrogen in the urine and as 1 g. of urinary nitrogen is associated with a loss of about 30 g. lean body mass it has been estimated that after major abdominal surgery an average man loses 300–450 g. of protein each day for 5–6 days.

Parenteral feeding of a combination of amino-acids and carbohydrate reduces the postoperative nitrogen loss and should be used when oral feeding cannot meet the total calorie requirements for more than a few days. The greater the delay in dealing with the catabolic response the more difficult it becomes to reverse the process and unchecked large amounts of muscle tissue are broken down. However, it is important to realize that parenteral feeding does not increase the rate of wound healing or speed up recovery of well-nourished patients after elective operations.

INDICATIONS FOR THE USE OF PARENTERAL FEEDING

i. Paralytic ileus.

ii. After some oesophageal and gastric operations. Many of these patients have lost up to 25 per cent of their body-weight prior to admission.

iii. Granulomatous disease of the large and small intestine with large alimentary losses of nitrogen.

iv. Enterocutaneous fistulae of the small intestine.

v. Unconscious patients in whom intestinal tube feeding has produced diarrhoea.

vi. Patients with severe burns.

The total calorie, protein, and fluid requirements for each patient must be assessed daily. For most patients 30–35 calories per kg. per day and 1·0–1·5 g. protein per kg. per day are sufficient to supply all the body's needs, but twice these amounts are often required after severe trauma and burns. The total calories are usually made up of a mixture of food substances as a marked excess of any particular one results in improper utilization of the materials. A rough guide to acceptable proportions of each foodstuff is:

Carbohydrate	50–70 per cent
Protein	10–15 per cent
Fat emulsions	20–40 per cent

PROTEIN

When given parenterally amino-acids can maintain the body's nitrogen balance and they are maximally utilized when their ratios are similar to those found in whole protein. With the exception of the dextrorotatory forms of methionine and phenylalanine the body can only utilize the laevorotatory forms of the amino-acids. These are given either as a protein hydrolysate or as prepared mixtures of synthetic amino-acids. Protein hydrolysates (Aminosol) are obtained by enzymatic hydrolysis of casein to form a mixture of laevorotatory amino-acids and simple polypeptides. Until recently only synthetic mixtures containing both the active laevorotatory and inactive dextrorotatory amino-acids (Trophysan) have been available but now pure synthetic laevorotatory preparations (Vamin, Aminoplex) are obtainable. The body requires calories to utilize the amino-acids and these must be infused at the same time; 200 calories are sufficient for each gramme of nitrogen but this may be as high as 300 calories in cases where there is evidence of excess catabolism or renal failure. The electrolyte content of amino-acid solutions can often be important as for example when the sodium content is high, fluid retention may occur.

CARBOHYDRATES

These readily available sources of calories are rapidly used by the body and do not give rise to toxic breakdown products. They have an antiketogenic action preserving the stores of protein in the body and protecting the liver from damage.

Glucose, as 10 per cent, 20 per cent, and 50 per cent

solutions, is the first choice but its utilization is dependent upon insulin.

Fructose is metabolized in the liver to form glycogen and is largely independent of insulin. Large concentrations of fructose should not be given to neonates or dehydrated patients as a severe metabolic acidosis may be induced by its conversion to lactate. It is available as 10 per cent and 20 per cent solutions.

Sorbitol is a sugar alcohol which is oxidized in the liver to fructose and can be used even when the liver is severely damaged. It is insulin independent but has the disadvantage of having a potent osmotic diuretic action which, following prolonged infusion, can produce an excessive loss of serum electrolytes. It is available as 20 per cent and 30 per cent solutions.

Ethyl alcohol is an important source of calories and although not a carbohydrate it is similar to these substances in its metabolism. It must not be given to patients with liver damage or in excess of 1 g. per kg. body-weight each day as liver damage has been reported with larger amounts; 2·5 per cent and 5 per cent solutions are used usually in combination with amino-acids and carbohydrates.

FATS

Enthusiasm for these substances varies as severely ill patients have great difficulty in their metabolism, and anaemia, weight-loss, and haemorrhage have been reported with their use. They are given as emulsions which consist of oil particles 0·5–1 μm. in diameter in water, an emulsifying agent and glucose, glycerin, or sorbitol to make the preparation isotonic. Fat is necessary in any prolonged intravenous feeding in order to prevent essential fatty acid deficiency.

Soya-bean oil (Intralipid) is generally accepted as being free from toxic side-effects, but when used over long periods is associated with the general problems of fats given parenterally. It is available as 10 per cent and 20 per cent emulsions.

Electrolyte solutions, drugs, or other solutions must not be added to infusion bottles containing fat emulsions. If a fat emulsion and a solution of amino-acids are to be given simultaneously separate infusion sets should be used and connected by a Y-tube so that mixing occurs only just before the fluids enter the circulation.

Preparations for parenteral feeding are shown in *Table* 7 and suitable régimes for their use are supplied by the distributors.

COMPLICATIONS OF PARENTERAL FEEDING

i. Phlebitis. Approximately 80 per cent of peripheral veins will develop thrombophlebitis if used for parenteral feeding longer than 2 days. Amino-acids and high concentrations of carbohydrate are extremely irritant and unfortunately the lower concentrations of carbohydrate do not provide sufficient calories, e.g., 1 litre of 5 per cent glucose provides only 200 calories; 10 and 20 per cent solutions of sorbitol cause little damage to peripheral veins and fat emulsions produce none at all. Phlebitis can be reduced by changing the infusion site in peripheral veins every day or by cannulating a large central vein at an early stage in the treatment.

ii. Toxic reactions. Both fat emulsions and casein hydrolysates can produce acute effects such as fever, backache, shivering, flushing, nausea, and headaches. If any of these effects are observed the infusion must be stopped and calories supplied by an alternative method.

iii. Routine blood analysis. A close check must be kept on the haemoglobin, serum electrolytes, and albumin levels. Intravenous feeding interferes with the estimation of these values and should be withheld for 4 hours before blood samples are taken.

iv. Patients with renal failure. For patients with renal failure a régime of 40 g. protein and 2000 calories of

Table 7. VALUES PER LITRE OF PARENTERAL FLUID

PREPARATION	MANUFACTURER	K-CALORIES	NITROGEN (g.)	CARBOHYDRATE (g.)	SODIUM (mmol.)	POTASSIUM (mmol.)	FAT (g.)
Protein mixtures							
Trophysan 10	Servier Laboratories	564	6·7	50	6	8	—
Trophysan-Lconc 10		724	13·1	100	10	8	—
Aminosol 10%	Kabi Vitrum Ltd	350	13·0	0	136	1·4	—
Aminosol-glucose		325	4·3	50	48	0·5	—
Aminosol Ethanol		900	4·3	150	48	0·5	—
Vamin fructose		650	9·4	100	50	20	—
glucose		650	9·4	100	50	20	—
'N'		250	9·4	0	50	20	—
Aminoplex 5	Geistich Sons Ltd	1000	5·0	125	35	15	—
Aminoplex 14		340	13·4	0	35	30	—
Aminofusin L600	Cambrian Chemicals Ltd	600	7·6	100	40	30	—
Aminofusin L1000		1000	7·6	100	40	30	—
Fat emulsions							
Intralipid 10%	Kabi Vitrum Ltd	1100	—	0	—	—	100
Intralipid 20%		2000	—	0	—	—	200
Carbohydrate solution							
Laevuflex	Geistlich Sons Ltd	820	—	200	—	—	—
Ethulose		980	—	150	—	—	—

carbohydrate reduces the breakdown of tissue protein and does not increase any rise in blood-urea. Fat must not be given immediately before haemodialysis as it sticks to the membranes and interferes with dialysis.

OSMOTIC DIURETICS

The intravenous administration of certain hypertonic solutions that are not metabolized in the body can produce a diuresis by increasing the osmotic pressure of the fluid in the renal tubules. These substances pass freely across the renal glomeruli and as they are not significantly reabsorbed in the tubules they are accompanied by decreased reabsorption of water, sodium, and chloride. They may be used in the prevention and treatment of oliguria or anuria and the treatment of refractory oedema, drug overdosage, cerebral oedema, and conditions with raised C.S.F. or intra-ocular pressures.

Urea and mannitol are most frequently employed, but in the past sucrose and hypertonic electrolyte solutions such as saline have been used with success. Oral urea (10–20 g. daily) is useful, but today it is usually given intravenously to produce an immediate effect. Mannitol is formed by the reduction of fructose and is available in 500-ml. packs of 10 per cent solution and 250-ml. packs of 20 or 25 per cent solutions which are infused over a period of 30–60 minutes. In patients with oliguria or anuria a test dose of mannitol 0·2 g. per kg. must be given over 3–5 minutes to assess the renal response. If it produces a renal output equivalent to 40 ml. urine per hour then the total dose can be given. If the kidneys do not respond to the test dose then impaired renal function can be assumed and no further mannitol should be given. Other contra-indications to its use are severe congestive heart failure, pregnancy, and metabolic oedema.

During treatment the general condition of the patient must be assessed repeatedly, all fluid intake and output measured and a careful check kept on the serum electrolytes. Patients under general anaesthesia or with a history of bladder outflow obstruction should be catheterized. If the recommended dose of mannitol is exceeded clinical signs of water intoxication, muscle rigidity, and pulmonary congestion can occur.

Chapter 10

S I (Système International)
Units and Normal Ranges

Since 1976 Pathology Departments will have been changing their method of reporting to use the metric system of
SI units. For a period of time both the conventional
system and SI units will be in use and the following
tables may help during the transition. The normal ranges
given are those in which 95 per cent of healthy adults
should fall, but must be taken as a general guide as differences with age and sex may be significant. Normal ranges
may also vary with the techniques used by different
laboratories and in these cases the laboratory may issue
appropriate tables.

For conversion from conventional to SI units a
conversion factor is given and its reciprocal value can be
used to convert back to conventional values. Concentration
of all substances, apart from haemoglobin, are expressed
as SI units per litre. This exception has been made as it
is expected that in the near future it will be possible to
express haemoglobin concentrations in molar terms, but
until then it will be expressed as g per dl.

Table 8. NAMES AND SYMBOLS OF SOME BASIC SI UNITS

QUANTITY	NAME OF UNIT	SYMBOL
Length	metre	m.
Mass	kilogram	kg.
Amount of substance	mole	mol.
Pressure	pascal	Pa.
Time	second	s.

Table 9. PREFIXES FOR SI UNITS

FACTOR	NAME	SYMBOL	FACTOR	NAME	SYMBOL
10^{12}	tera	T	10^{-1}	deci	d
10^{9}	giga	G	10^{-2}	centi	c
10^{6}	mega	M	10^{-3}	milli	m
10^{3}	kilo	k	10^{-6}	micro	μ
10^{2}	hecto	h	10^{-9}	nano	n
10^{1}	deca	da	10^{-12}	pico	p

Table 10. NORMAL RANGES OF VALUES

Key to symbols: B = blood; P = plasma; S = serum.

		CONVENTIONAL UNITS	SI UNITS	CONVERSION FACTOR
a. Haematological (B)				
Hb	male	13.5–18.0 g./dl.	13.5–18.0 g./dl.	None
	female	11.5–16.5 g./dl.	11.5–16.5 g./dl.	None
P.C.V.	male	40–54%	0.40–0.54	0.01
	female	35–47%	0.35–0.47	0.01
M.C.H.C.		32–36%	32–36 g./dl.	None
M.C.H.		27–32 $\mu\mu$g.	27–32 pg.	None
M.C.V.		76–96 μm.^{3}	76–96 fl.	None
R.B.Cs.	male	4.5–6.5×10^6/mm.^{3}	4.5–6.5×10^{12}/l.	None
	female	3.9–5.6×10^6/mm.^{3}	3.9–5.6×10^{12}/l.	None
W.B.Cs.		4–10×10^3/mm.^{3}	4–10×10^9/l.	None
Platelets		150–400×10^3/mm.^{3}	150–400×10^9/l.	None
Reticulocytes		0.2–2.0%	0.2–2.0%	None
b. Biochemical				
Bilirubin	S	<1.0 mg./100 ml.	<17 μmol./l.	17.1
Calcium	S	8.5–10.5 mg./100 ml.	2.1–2.6 mmol./l.	0.25
Chloride	P	95–105 mEq./l.	95–105 mmol./l.	None
Cholesterol	S	140–240 mg./100 ml.	3.6–7.2 mmol./l.	0.0259
Creatinine	P	0.7–1.4 mg./100 ml.	60–120 μmol./l.	88.4
Iron,	male S	80–180 μg./100 ml.	14–32 μmol./l.	0.179
	female S	60–160 μg./100 ml.	11–29 μmol./l.	0.179
Iron-binding capacity	S	250–400 μg./100 ml.	45–72 μmol./l.	0.179
Magnesium	P	1.8–2.2 mg./100 ml.	0.7–0.9 mmol./l.	0.411
Protein: total	S	6.0–8.2 g./100 ml.	60–82 g./l.	10

		CONVENTIONAL UNITS	SI UNITS	CONVERSION FACTOR
albumin	S	3·6-5·2 g./100 ml.	36-52 g./l.	10
globulin	S	2·1-3·7 g./100 ml.	21-37 g./l.	10
Phosphorus	P	2·4-4·2 mg./100 ml.	0·8-1·4 mmol./l.	0·323
Potassium	P	3·5-5·0 mEq./l.	3·5-5·0 mmol./l.	None
Sodium	P	134-148 mEq./l.	134-148 mmol./l.	None
Urea	P	<40 mg./100 ml.	<6·6 mmol./l.	0·166
c. Acid-base parameters				
PCO_2	B	31-45 mm.Hg	4·1-6·0 kPa.	0·133
Std HCO_3	B	21-31 mEq./l.	21-31 mmol./l.	None
Base excess	B	±3 mEq./l.	±3 mmol./l.	None
PO_2	B	80-110 mm.Hg	10·5-14·5 kPa.	0·133
Total CO_2	P	22-28 mEq./l.	22-28 mmol./l.	None
d. Other blood values				
Glucose: fasting	B	65-95 mg./100 ml.	3·6-5·3 mmol./l.	0·0555
Random	B	65-175 mg./100 ml.	3·6-9·7 mmol./l.	0·0555
e. Urine values				
Calcium		100-300 mg./24 hours	2·5-7·5 mmol./24 hours	0·025
Creatinine		1000-2000 mg./24 hours	9-18 mmol./24 hours	8·84
Potassium		40-140 mEq./l.	40-140 mmol./l.	None
Sodium		100-250 mEq./l.	100-250 mmol./l.	None

Chapter 11

Drugs in common use for surgical emergencies

The penicillins are bactericidal and act by interfering with the formation of the bacterial cell wall. Cross-sensitivity occurs to all the penicillins and superinfection with *Proteus, Pseudomonas,* and *candida* may occur. Staphylococcal enterocolitis and systemic mycotic disease are serious complications of oral therapy.

DOSES FOR CHILDREN

Although there are several methods for calculating suitable doses for infants and children, Gaubius' method is both easy to remember and quite efficient.

	Fraction of the adult dose
Under 1 year:	$\frac{1}{12}$
Under 2 years:	$\frac{1}{8}$
Under 3 years:	$\frac{1}{6}$
Under 4 years:	$\frac{1}{4}$
Under 7 years:	$\frac{1}{3}$
Under 14 years:	$\frac{1}{2}$
Under 20 years:	$\frac{2}{3}$

Table 1

NAME	PROPRIETARY NAME	ACTION	INDICATIONS
Phenoxymethyl-penicillin (penicillin V)	Crystapen V, etc.		Cocci and some Gram-negative bacilli
Benzylpenicillin	Crystalline penicillin G		
Ampicillin	Penbritin Amfipen	Broad spectrum	*Strep. faecalis*; *E. coli*; some *Proteus*; Salmonellae
Methicillin	Celebenin	Not affected by staphylococcal penicillinase	Resistant staphylococci
Cloxacillin	Orbenin		
Carbenicillin	Pyopen	Not affected by penicillinase of some strains of *Proteus*, *Pseudomonas*, and coliforms	*P. pyocanea*; *Proteus*; *E. coli*.
Streptomycin		Rapidly bactericidal Should not be given alone as organisms soon become resistant	Gram-negative organisms; mycobacteria; broad-spectrum when given with penicillin
Tetracycline Oxytetracycline	Too numerous to mention	Bacteriostatic	Broad-spectrum an mixed infections

Antibiotics

| AMOUNT | DOSAGE | | COMPLICATIONS | CONTRA-INDICATIONS |
	ROUTE	FREQUENCY		
250 mg.	Oral	4–6 hours	Hypersensitivity and anaphylactic reactions	
·5–2 mega-units	i.m., i.v.	4–6 hours		
250 mg.–1 g.	Oral, i.m.; i.v.	6 hours	Diarrhoea; skin rashes	
g.	i.m.	4–6 hours	Injections are painful	
00 mg.	Oral;	4–6 hours		
50 mg.	i.m.	4–6 hours		
–30 g.	Continuous i.v. infusion	Daily	Resistant strains quickly emerge if dosage is insufficient. Excreted in the urine, so probenecid 1 g. t.d.s. orally is also given	
·5 g.	i.m.	Twice daily for 5 days	Dermatitis; allergy; resistance; eighth nerve damage	Myasthenia gravis
50–500 mg.	Oral	6 hours	Intestinal discomfort and diarrhoea; stomatitis; delays bone growth and discolours unerupted teeth; moniliasis; cross-resistance is common	Impaired renal or hepatic function; pregnancy Children up to 12 years of age. Administration with milk, antacids or mineral supplements containing salts of calcium, magnesium or iron.
00 mg.	i.m.	6 hours		

Table 11

NAME	PROPRIETARY NAME	ACTION	INDICATIONS
Chloramphenicol	Chloromycetin; Clorcetin; Kemicetine	Bacteriostatic	Broad-spectrum; severe infections where other antibiotics may not be effective, e.g., faecal peritonitis
Erythyromycin	Erycen; Erythrocin; Erythromid; Ilotycin; Ilosone	Primarily bacteriostatic with some bactericidal action	Gram-negative organisms
Cephaloridine*	Ceporin	Bactericidal; not affected by staphylococcal penicillinase	Gram-positive bacteriaemia
Kanamycin*	Kannasyn; Kantrex	Bactericidal	Broad-spectrum; Gram-negative bacteriaemia
Gentamicin*	Cidomycin; Genticin	Bactericidal	Bacteriaemia due to *Proteus*, *Pseudomonas*, *pyocyanea* or *E. coli*
Colistin sulphomethate*	Colomycin		Gram-negative infections; *Pseudomonas*
Lincomycin	Lincocin; Mycivin	Bactericidal or bacteriostatic depending on concentration	Gram-positive organisms; Bacteroides
Clindamycin	Dalacin C		

* Doses of these drugs must be modified for age, body-weight, and physical state.

Continued

	DOSAGE		COMPLICATIONS	CONTRA-INDICATIONS
AMOUNT	ROUTE	FREQUENCY		
500 mg.	Oral	6 hours for 5–7 days	Dryness of the mouth; nausea, vomiting; diarrhoea; bone-marrow depression; blood dyscrasias (rare)	Should not be used with anticoagulants, anticonvulsants, or hypoglycaemic agents
500 mg.	s.c.; i.m.; i.v.	6 hours		
250–500 mg.	Oral	6 hours	Nausea; vomiting; diarrhoea; pruritus; resistant strains of staphylococci emerge rapidly	
500 mg.	i.m.	6 hours	Allergies; skin rashes; resistance	Renal tubular necrosis
250 mg.	i.m.	6 hours	Eighth nerve damage; nephrotoxic; resistance	Renal impairment; neonates; pregnancy; the use of other ototoxic drugs
50 mg.	i.m.	8 hours		
10,000 units per kg. every 24 hours	i.m.	Divided doses	Paraesthesia	
500 mg.–1g.	Oral	8 hours	Diarrhoea; colitis; abdominal cramps; vomiting; skin rashes	Pre-existing monilial infection; Hypersensitivity; allergies; Pregnancy; neonates; liver or renal disease
500 mg.	i.v.	8–12 hours		
500 mg.	i.m.	12–24 hours		
150–450 mg.	Oral	6 hours		

Table 12.

NAME	PROPRIETARY NAME	ACTION	INDICATIONS FOR USE
Aspirin		Raises the threshold of somatic pain without reducing the reaction to pain. Antipyretic	Mild pain of somatic origin. Musculoskeletal pain; pyrexia
Paracetamol	Calpol; Panadol; Tabalgin, etc.		
Codeine		Raises the threshold of pain perception and reduces the reaction to pain sensation. Morphine and diamorphine both stimulate and depress the medullary centres	Moderate pain
Dihydrocodeine	D.F. 118; Paracodin		
Pentazocine	Fortral		Severe pain
Pethidine			
Morphine			Severe pain; relief of anxiety by producing euphoria
Diamorphine	Heroin		

ANALGESICS

DOSAGE			COMPLICATIONS	CONTRA-INDICATIONS
AMOUNT	ROUTE	FREQUENCY		
0·3–1 g.	Oral	6 hours	Indigestion; haematemesis; asthma; urticaria	Peptic ulceration
0·5–1 g.	Oral	6 hours		
10–60 mg.	Oral	4–6 hours	Constipation; nausea; giddiness	Depressed liver function; asthma
30–60 mg.	Oral with food	4–6 hours		
50 mg.	i.m.	4–6 hours		
50–100 mg.	Oral	3–4 hours		Renal, liver, and respiratory depression; mono-amine oxidase inhibitors; pregnancy
30–60 mg.	i.m.	3–4 hours		
50–100 mg.	Oral or i.m.	4 hours	Dizziness; nausea; sweating; tolerance	
25–50 mg.	i.v.	4 hours		
10–20 mg.	s.c.; i.m.	4 hours	Depression of respiration, nausea; vomiting; smooth-muscle contraction; tolerance	Circulatory shock
5–10 mg.	s.c.; i.m.	4 hours		

Table 13.

NAME	PROPRIETARY NAME	ACTION	INDICATIONS FOR USE
Atropine		Relaxation of smooth muscle and inhibition of endothelial secretions	The relief of smooth-muscle colics and to dry up endothelial secretions
Propantheline	Aclobrom; Pro-Banthine		

Table 14.

NAME	PROPRIETARY NAME	ACTION	INDICATIONS FOR USE
Heparin	Pularin	Inhibits the activation of prothrombin and neutralizes thrombin	Immediate anticoagulation. Dose regulated according to the clotting time. It should be maintained between 10 and 15 minutes
Phenindione	Dindevan	Antagonism of vitamin K and depression of prothrombin formation but takes 12–24 hours to become effective	Maintenance of anticoagulation; the doses are regulated according to the prothrombin activity of the blood
Warfarin	Marevan; W.B. Warfarin		

Antispasmodics

DOSAGE			COMPLICATIONS	CONTRA-INDICATIONS
AMOUNT	ROUTE	FREQUENCY		
0·25–2·00 mg.	s.c.; i.m.; i.v.	4–6 hours	Blurring of vision and a dry mouth	Glaucoma; prostatic enlargement; pyloric stenosis
15 mg.	Oral	8 hours or before meals		
15 mg.	s.c.; i.m.; i.v.	6 hours		

Anticoagulants

DOSAGE			COMPLICATIONS	CONTRA-INDICATIONS
AMOUNT	ROUTE	FREQUENCY		
10,000 units initially	i.v.	4–6 hours	Bleeding	Bleeding diatheses and conditions, e.g., peptic ulcers; liver and renal disease; uncontrolled hypertension; subacute bacterial endocarditis; pregnancy
200–300 mg. initial oral dose. Then 25–100 mg. daily				
30–50 mg. initial oral dose. No more for 2 days, then 3–10 mg. daily				

Table 15.

NAME	PROPRIETARY NAME	ACTION	INDICATIONS FOR USE
Digoxin	Lanoxin	Increases the force of contraction of the myocardium; depresses conduction through the heart. The actions are increased by potassium depletion which may produce toxic effects	Congestive heart failure; atrial fibrillation
Digitoxin			
Lanatoside-C	Cedilanid		

DIGITALIS GLYCOSIDES

DOSAGE			COMPLICATIONS	CONTRA-INDICATIONS
AMOUNT	ROUTE	FREQUENCY		
Initial dose 1–1·5 mg.	Oral; i.m.; i.v.	Single dose	Headache; anorexia; nausea; vomiting; bradycardia; ventricular extrasystoles; coupling of pulse	Potassium depletion
Maintenance dose 0·25 mg.	Oral; i.m.	1–3 times a day		
Initial dose 1–1·5 mg.	Oral; i.m.; i.v.	Single dose		
Maintenance dose 0·25–0·20 mg.	Oral; i.m.	Daily		
Initial dose 1–1·5 mg.	Oral; i.m.; i.v.	Single dose		
Maintenance dose 0·25 mg.	Oral; i.m.	1–4 times a day		

Table 16.

NAME	PROPRIETARY NAME	ACTION	INDICATIONS FOR USE
Benzo-thiadiazines			
a. Chlorothiazide	Saluric	Increases the excretion of sodium, chloride, and water by the kidneys. As potassium is also lost 2–3 g. KCl are given daily for replacement. Potentiates the action of some hypotensive agents	Fluid retention; hypertension
b. Hydrochloro-thiazide	Direma; Esidrex; Hydro saluric		
c. Hydro-flumethiazide	Hydrenox; Naclex		
d. Bendrofluazide	Aprinox; Berkozide; Centyl; Neo-Naclex		
Frusemide	Lasix	As above but less potassium loss	As above. When a speedy diuresis is required
Spironolactone	Aldactone-A	Antagonism of aldosterone. Must be given with one of the above	Oedema resistant to conventional diuretics; cirrhosis; nephrotic syndrome

DIURETICS

DOSAGE			COMPLICATIONS	CONTRA-INDICATIONS
AMOUNT	ROUTE	FREQUENCY		
0·5–2·0 g.	Oral	Daily	Allergic reactions; potassium depletion; blood dyscrasias	Severe renal or hepatic dysfunction
25–100 mg.	Oral	Daily		
25–100 mg.	Oral	Daily		
5–10 mg.	Oral	Daily		
40–120 mg.	Oral	Daily or alternate days	Potassium depletion	Acute glomerulonephritis; anuria or acute renal failure; gross liver damage
20–40 mg.	i.m., i.v.	1–3 times a day		
25–50 mg.	Oral	1–4 times a day		Anuria; severe liver damage

Table 17

NAME	PROPRIETARY NAME	ACTION	INDICATIONS FOR USE
Vitamin C		Assists healing	Major operations, particularly in the elderly patient
Vitamin K	Aquamephyton; Konakion; Synkavit	Formation of prothrombin in the liver	Reversal of anticoagulant-induced prothrombin deficiency; jaundice
Vitamin B complex with vitamin C	Parentrovite		Confusional episodes following severe illness

VITAMINS

	DOSAGE		COMPLICATIONS	CONTRA-INDICATIONS
AMOUNT	ROUTE	FREQUENCY		
oo mg.	Oral	6 hours		
o mg.	i.m.	Daily		
< 50 mg.	i.v.	Single dose		
a) High potency paired ampoules	i.m.; i.v.	Daily		
b) Maintenance paired ampoules	i.m.	Daily		

Index